Chi Kung
for Women's Health
and Sexual Vitality

Chi Kung
for Women's Health
and Sexual Vitality

A Handbook of Simple Exercises and Techniques

Mantak Chia
and William U. Wei

Destiny Books
Rochester, Vermont • Toronto, Canada

Destiny Books
One Park Street
Rochester, Vermont 05767
www.DestinyBooks.com

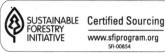

Text stock is SFI certified

Destiny Books is a division of Inner Traditions International

Originally published in Thailand in 2012 by Universal Tao Publications under the title *Uterus Chi Kung: Techniques and Exercises for Uterus Cancer Prevention and Sexual Vitality*

Library of Congress Cataloging-in-Publication Data
Chia, Mantak, 1944–
  Chi kung for women's health and sexual vitality : a handbook of simple exercises and techniques / Mantak Chia and William U. Wei.
    pages cm
  Includes bibliographical references and index.
  ISBN 978-1-62055-225-4 (pbk.) — ISBN 978-1-62055-226-1 (e-book)
  1. Women—Health and hygiene. 2. Gynecology. 3. Reproductive health. 4. Qi gong. I. Wei, William U. II. Title.
  RG121.C57 2013
  618.1—dc23

                                                                        2013044943

Printed and bound in the United States by Lake Book Manufacturing, Inc.
The text stock is SFI certified. The Sustainable Forestry Initiative® program promotes sustainable forest management.

10 9 8 7 6 5 4 3 2 1

Text design by Priscilla Baker and layout by Debbie Glogover
This book was typeset in Garamond Premier Pro with Present and Futura Std as display typefaces

Illustrations by Udon Jandee
Photographs by Sopitnapa Promnon

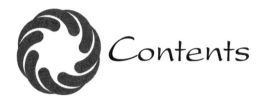 Contents

Acknowledgments

The Universal Healing Tao publications staff involved in the preparation and production of *Chi Kung for Women's Health and Sexual Vitality* extend our gratitude to the many generations of Taoist masters who have passed on their special lineage, in the form of an unbroken oral transmission, over thousands of years. We thank Taoist Master I Yun (Yi Eng) for his openness in transmitting the formulas of Taoist Inner Alchemy.

We offer our eternal gratitude to our parents and teachers for their many gifts to us. Remembering them brings joy and satisfaction to our continued efforts in presenting the Universal Healing Tao system. As always, their contribution has been crucial in presenting the concepts and techniques of the Universal Healing Tao.

We wish to thank the thousands of unknown men and women of the Chinese healing arts who developed many of the methods and ideas presented in this book. We offer our gratitude to Bob Zuraw for sharing his kindness, healing techniques, and Taoist understandings.

We thank the many contributors essential to this book's final form: the editorial and production staff at Inner Traditions/Destiny Books for their efforts to clarify the text and produce a handsome new edition of the book and Nancy Yeilding for her line edit of the new edition.

We also wish to thank Colin Drown, Matthew Koren, Otto Thamboon, our senior instructors Wilbert and Saumya Wils, and Charles Morris for their editorial work on the earlier edition of this book. A special thanks goes to our Thai production team: Hirunyathorn Punsan, Sopitnapa Promnon, Udon Jandee, and Suthisa Chaisam.

Putting Chi Kung for Women's Health and Sexual Vitality into Practice

The practices described in this book have been used successfully for thousands of years by Taoists trained by personal instruction. Readers should not undertake the practice without receiving personal transmission and training from a certified instructor of the Universal Healing Tao, since certain of these practices, if done improperly, may cause injury or result in health problems. This book is intended to supplement individual training by the Universal Healing Tao and to serve as a reference guide for these practices. Anyone who undertakes these practices on the basis of this book alone does so entirely at her own risk.

The meditations, practices, and techniques described herein are not intended to be used as an alternative or substitute for professional medical treatment and care. If any readers are suffering from illnesses based on mental or emotional disorders, an appropriate professional health care practitioner or therapist should be consulted. Such problems should be corrected before you start training.

Neither the Universal Healing Tao nor its staff and instructors can be responsible for the consequences of any practice or misuse of the information contained in this book. If the reader undertakes any exercise without strictly following the instructions, notes, and warnings, the responsibility must lie solely with the reader.

This book does not attempt to give any medical diagnosis, treatment, prescription, or remedial recommendation in relation to any human disease, ailment, suffering, or physical condition whatsoever.

Introduction

After over fifty years of sharing Chi Kung daily practices for women's health through the Universal Healing Tao system, we find it hard to believe that 60 percent of women after the age of thirty suffer from some form of gynecological malfunctioning or cancer, which can lead ultimately to death. The simple techniques of Chi Kung for women enable every woman to literally get in touch with her urogenital area and eliminate such problems and discomforts by just simply touching herself with the proper intentions. At the suggestion of Ehud Sperling, the publisher of Inner Traditions/Destiny Books, we have gathered together in this book a series of Universal Healing Tao techniques and daily exercises that will support the health of the female reproductive system and sexual vitality.

Cancer is the uncontrolled growth of abnormal cells, which feed off the body to maintain this growth. When a cell is damaged or altered without repair to its system, it usually dies. However, cancer cells, also termed malignant cells or tumor cells, proliferate and a mass of cells develops. Many cancers and the abnormal cells that compose the cancer tissue are further identified by the name of the tissue that the cells originate from, such as lung cancer, breast cancer, uterine cancer, or colon cancer.

There are five main types of cancer that affect a woman's reproductive organs: cervical, ovarian, uterine, vaginal, and vulvar. As a group, they are referred to as gynecologic cancer. (A sixth type of gynecologic cancer is the very rare fallopian tube cancer.) Uterine cancer is the fourth most common cancer in women in the United States and it is the most commonly diagnosed gynecologic cancer. All women are at risk for uterine cancer, and the risk increases with age. Uterine cancer usually occurs during or after menopause. The risk is increased by obesity and by taking estrogen-alone hormone replacement therapy (also called menopausal hormone therapy). Each year, approximately 35,000 women in the United States get uterine cancer.

The symptoms of uterine cancer include unusual vaginal bleeding or discharge, trouble urinating, pelvic pain, and pain during intercourse. Generally, the tumor grows slowly and remains confined to the area for many years. During this time, the tumor produces little or no symptoms or outward signs (abnormalities on physical examination). However, all uterine cancers do not behave similarly. Some aggressive types of uterine cancer grow and spread more rapidly than others and can cause a significant shortening of life expectancy in women affected by them. A trained pathologist observing uterus biopsy specimens under the microscope can calculate a measure of uterine cancer. As the cancer advances, however, it can spread beyond the uterus into the surrounding tissues. Moreover, the cancer also can metastasize, spreading throughout other areas of the body, such as the bones, lungs, and liver. Symptoms and signs, therefore, are more often associated with advanced uterine cancer.

When uterine cancer is found early, treatment is most effective. Treatment varies depending on your overall health, how advanced the cancer is, and whether hormones affect its growth. Many low-risk tumors can be safely followed with active surveillance. Through conventional medicine, curative treatment generally involves surgery, various forms of radiation therapy, or, less commonly, cryosurgery; hormonal therapy and chemotherapy are generally reserved for cases of advanced disease. The age and underlying health of the woman, the extent of metastasis, appearance under the microscope, and response of the cancer to initial treatment are important in determining the outcome of the disease. The decision whether or not to treat localized uterine cancer with curative intent is a patient trade-off between the expected beneficial and harmful effects in terms of patient survival and quality of life.

Food and sex are humankind's greatest appetites. From a Taoist's point of view they also offer opportunities for our greatest healing exercises, if we have the proper understanding of how use them to heal our bodies. From the Universal Healing Tao system, as demonstrated in the Destiny Books editions of several Universal Healing Tao publications— particularly *Healing Love through the Tao, Bone Marrow Nei Kung, Cosmic Detox,* and *Cosmic Nutrition*—we have assembled a sequence of Chi Kung for women daily practices that will balance and maintain the sexual organs, while rejuvenating your sexual vitality.

The internal egg exercises, genital massage techniques, and Chi Weight Lifting are all aspects of what is known in the Universal Tao system as Bone Marrow Nei Kung. *Nei Kung* means "practicing with your internal power," and Bone Marrow Nei Kung is a Taoist art of self-cultivation that employs mental and physical techniques to rejuvenate the bone marrow, thereby enhancing the blood and nourishing the life force within.

Bone Marrow Nei Kung overlaps with three primary Taoist approaches to sexual energy: Healing Love, Sexual Energy Massage, and Chi Weight Lifting. These three methods are used to increase sexual energy and hormones in the body, providing the means to achieve great personal power and health.

The Healing Love practices enable a person to retain sexual energy, stimulate the brain, and rejuvenate the organs and glands to increase the production of Ching Chi (sexual energy). The techniques reverse the usual outward flow of sexual energy during the orgasmic phase of sex, and draw the Ching Chi upward into the body, thereby enhancing internal healing capabilities. The release of Ching Chi into the body through the Sexual Energy Massage or Chi Weight Lifting methods presupposes that it is already abundant within the sexual center. If one suffers from weakened kidneys or any internal dysfunctions, the Healing Love methods should be mastered to accumulate Ching Chi before attempting the other two methods.

In this book, exercises derived from the Healing Love practice are used as nonsexual techniques that help to rejuvenate the internal organs and glands with sexual energy. The Healing Love practices of Ovarian Breathing, Ovarian Compression, and the Power Lock can be found in chapter 1, "Exercises for the Female Reproductive System."

While Healing Love prevents the loss of Ching Chi and rejuvenates the internal system, the Sexual Energy Massage, presented in chapter 2, releases higher concentrations of Ching Chi into the body for cultivating the bone marrow and stimulating the endocrine glands. Chapter 2 also presents the Internal Egg Exercise, which strengthens the sexual region and aids the transformation of raw sexual energy into life-force energy. When used together, the two practices constitute a safer method of disseminating sexual energy than Chi Weight Lifting.

Chi Weight Lifting, presented in chapter 3, is the ultimate practice for releasing sexual energy into the body. Its practice provides the greatest abundance of Ching Chi for healing and rejuvenation. It also releases maximum quantities of sexual hormones, which stimulate the pituitary gland to prevent aging. In addition, the technique exercises the fascial connections between the sexual and other internal organs, thereby strengthening the organs and glands.

However, Chi Weight Lifting is an advanced practice and should not be attempted without the proper training. After having received Universal Tao instruction, a student may proceed with caution to lift light weights attached to a stone egg held in the vaginal canal. At this level, the Sexual Energy Massage is used before and after Chi Weight Lifting, first to prepare the genitals, and afterward to replenish the circulation in the sexual center.

A woman's health and her sexual vitality are also supported by proper nutrition and thorough cleansing of the body, especially its "front and back doors." These topics are covered in chapter 4.

Chapter 5 offers a summary version of all of the exercises, for your ready reference.

All of these practices will aid you in breaking up any energetic blockages in the pelvic region, opening up the energetic pathways, and preserving optimum gynecologic health, supporting sexual vitality and your ability to maintain your sexual life well into advanced age without discomfort, pain, or malfunction.

Exercises for the Female Reproductive System

In the East, as well as in the West, exercise is a crucial way to keep the body healthy. But when it comes to increasing sexual energy, the teachers of the East have taken exercise to a new level. To strengthen sexual energy, and thus strengthen the senses and the whole body, the Eastern traditions have developed exercises that focus specifically on the sexual area. In the Tao, sexual exercises are not merely a way to enhance sexual pleasure or become more attractive. These exercises are a means to enjoy a more vigorous and healthy body, a way to become sensitive to deeper and more intense emotions, and to cultivate spiritual energy.

The sexual area is the root of an individual's health. Leading into the pelvis are a vast number of nerve endings and channels for the veins and arteries. Here are located tissues that communicate with every square inch of the body. All of the major acupuncture meridians that carry energy to the vital organs pass by this area. If it is blocked or weak, energy will dissipate and the organs and brain will suffer. This is what happens to many people in old age. As their rectal and pelvic muscles sag and become loose, their vital chi energy slowly drains out, leaving them weak and feeble. Strength in this region is of inestimable importance.

CULTIVATING OVARIAN POWER

The ancient Taoists had extraordinarily astute powers of observation, and their findings on the subject of sex are surprisingly consistent among different groups and over long stretches of time, which in China means not hundreds but thousands of years. This is significant because many groups did not know of any others' abilities, whereabouts, or even existence, since these esoteric practices were kept very secret.

The ancient Taoists noted that the ovaries, as the factories that produce sexual energy in the form of eggs and female hormones, are of prime importance, because all of the vital organs, such as the brain, must contribute some of their own reserves to create and maintain them. It is said that anatomy is destiny: women are designed to be mothers. A baby girl's ovaries are immature, small, and smooth, but they contain the power necessary to create the three to five hundred eggs she will produce in her reproductive years, plus a reserve of potentially 450,000 eggs. In any case, whether a woman has children or not, her body continues cyclically to produce ovary energy. Instead of wasting that energy, it can be conserved through transformation into another form for later use.

The Taoist exercises given in this chapter—Ovarian Breathing and Ovarian and Vaginal Compression—provide a way to use that ovarian power. The Ovarian Breathing exercise will help you to open and utilize the channels of the Microcosmic Orbit, which runs from the sexual center up the spine to the crown, then down the front of the body and back to the navel. (See chapter 5 for instructions on opening the Microcosmic Orbit.) In Ovarian Breathing you use your mind to draw the warm, yang, vital egg energy up the spine to your head and to the third eye (located mid-eyebrow), down through the tongue (raised up to the palate), the heart, the solar plexus, finally to be stored in the navel. You will be drawing on the energy generated by the ovaries, eggs, and hormones themselves. At first the process is slow, but later a simple thought will send delightful waves of energy up your back to your head.

Crucial to the ability to control this flow of sexual energy is the strength of a group of muscles we refer to as the "Chi Muscle." The Chi

Muscle consists of the PC or pubococcygeus muscle (which stretches from the pubic bone to the coccyx or tailbone, forming the floor of the pelvic cavity), the muscles of the pelvic and urogenital diaphragms, the sphincter muscle of the anus, and many involuntary muscles located in the perineum region (see also figure 3.1 of chapter 3). The second exercise, Ovarian Compression, trains you to have more control of the Chi Muscle to build up warm Ching Chi in the ovaries and to move this energy safely upward.

A Woman's Menstrual Cycle

Most women have a profound connection with their menstrual cycles. Women students of the Universal Tao system have revealed how sensitive they are to what seem to be subtle changes in their cycles. They notice right away if their periods are one day early or late, if they last a day longer or are a day shorter, and whether the consistency or color of discharge varies from what they have come to expect. Many women even remember an event that occurred the day they received their first periods. Those memories may be pleasant or unpleasant, but they remain indelible. One woman remembers the day as the first time a man tried to pick her up; another remembers that her mother slapped her face (a gesture of welcome into the world of being a woman). Yet another woman hit a home run in a softball game that day.

On the other hand, for many women, the menstrual cycle becomes a source of confusion and uncertainty. They are unsure about fertile times, are ashamed of secretions and odors, are discontent with available birth control methods, develop anger at common childbirth practices, or harbor a simultaneous dependency on and distrust of the medical profession.

Some women go through life with few problems with their cycles, having easy periods, uncomplicated births, and smooth transitions into menopause. Others have distressing problems, such as recurrent vaginal infections, abnormal Pap smears, difficult births, or hysterectomies, or may take synthetic hormones because of disabling hot flashes during menopause. Major changes can occur in the menstrual cycles as well as in many other aspects in the lives of some women simply by practicing Ovarian Breathing.

If You Practice Celibacy

No matter who you are, sexual energy is constantly building up and accumulating in the sexual region. Some negative evidence about the health of celibates has been collected, based on studies of priests and nuns who use only willpower to suppress the sexual fire within. This evidence suggests that the practice of celibacy by women has brought on the eventual deterioration of the sexual organs due to long-term congestion in the ovaries or breasts, which in turn affects the internal organs.

Some celibates are able to transform their sexual energy naturally, and as a result no problems arise in the celibate state. A woman who is not so naturally enlightened will find an accumulation of too much sexual energy in her body and sexual organs. This energy tends to need a release, and if the woman has no way to handle the problem properly, the energy can affect her adversely, multiplying her negative emotions. Without properly cultivating sexual energy and opening the energy channels between the lower and upper body, the sexual energy is blocked, thereby congesting blood and hormones in the woman's genitals, ovaries, and cervix. A celibate woman can avoid such problems by practicing Ovarian Breathing and other Healing Love techniques (which can be found in detail in *Healing Love through the Tao,* Destiny Books, 2005).

Yang Energy and the Menstrual Cycle

There are three distinct parts to the menstrual cycle. First is the menstrual period itself. Then, after menstruation, an ovary spurts several immature eggs into action, and usually one egg matures completely. Surrounded by a jelly-like covering, it breaks out of the ovary. Third, after ovulation, the ruptured area of the ovary heals and forms the corpus luteum, or yellow body. This yellow body produces progesterone. The function of progesterone is to keep the uterine lining from sloughing off. If the egg unites with a sperm and a pregnancy starts, progesterone will be secreted during the entire pregnancy. If there is no fertilization, the ovary will produce a spurt of estrogen, and the menstruation cycle will begin.

Ancient records point out that in the first part of a woman's cycle, a

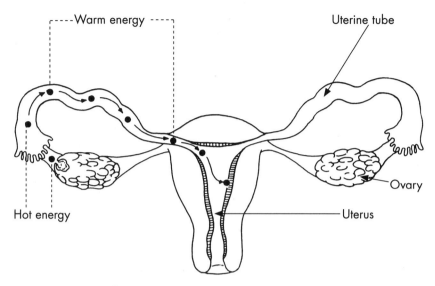

Fig. 1.1. Energy of ovulation: During the first stages of ovulation the energy is hot. As the egg travels toward the uterus, the energy turns warm.

tremendous storage of hot life-force energy, which they called yang Ching Chi (Ovarian Chi), takes place (fig. 1.1). During a woman's ovulation, yang energy activates and charges an egg with full potential life force; this is a sign of a strong and youthful energy with the power to create and heal.

As the woman's cycle continues and the egg moves out of the body, the experience of heat gives way to what has been described as a mildly warm quality. All sexual energy, whether male or female, is yin in its latent or resting state. At this time the aroused sexual energy is more yin in nature, thus it is more healing than creative. It is important to use this sexual energy and not let its vitality pour outward.

Ovarian Chi, or Ching Chi, is denser than the life force, or chi, that normally circulates in the Microcosmic Orbit. Since it is thicker and slower to move, this energy needs all the help it can get to move upward to a higher energy center. Therefore it is important to be sure the channel of the Microcosmic Orbit is open and the chi is flowing before proceeding to Ovarian Breathing. Then the more you can bring the Ching Chi (sexual energy) upward, the more you will heal and revitalize as it travels through the channel in its loop up the spine to the head and down the front through the navel, genitals, and perineum, linking the various organs and glands with each other and with the brain. This energy can also be used to heal and revitalize your partner.

The Taoists note, and women's experiences to date confirm, that the part of the cycle between menstruation and ovulation is the time that a woman will receive the maximum benefit from the practice of Ovarian Breathing, with continued practice then being optional until the next cycle. The process of Ovarian Breathing will draw energy out of the egg. Imagine having access to an energy that is powerful enough to bestow life!

In Taoism, cultivation of the movement of the pelvis, perineum, urogenital diaphragm, anus, and the sacral and cranial pumps is very important and necessary in helping to move the sexual energy up the spine.

The Body's Diaphragms

The body possesses not one but several diaphragms. Everyone is familiar with the thoracic diaphragm in the chest, which separates the heart and lungs from the abdominal organs and helps us breathe. When you inhale, this diaphragm lowers, thus increasing the space in the chest and allowing the lungs to fill. The deeper the breath, the lower the diaphragm moves.

Less is known about the pelvic and urogenital diaphragms, which separate the pelvis from the perineum. True breathing comes from these lower diaphragms. They are an exceedingly important element in the Taoist practice of transmitting the energy generated from the sexual organs into a higher energy form. They serve as floodgates, opening to spurt energy to the organs, or as pistons, pumping the energy up to higher centers. To practice Ovarian Breathing properly, you must use not only the chest diaphragm, but also the pelvic and urogenital diaphragms (fig. 1.2).

The Pelvic Diaphragm

The pelvic diaphragm is a muscular wall that extends across the lower part of the torso. It is suspended between the pubic symphysis (pubic bones) in front and the coccyx (at the bottom of the spine) in back (fig. 1.3). Several organs penetrate this muscular partition as it lies between the pelvic cavity and the perineum. These organs are the urethra, the vagina, and the rectum. One function of the pelvic diaphragm is to support these organs. Therefore, control over this diaphragm provides you with greater control over these organs. The pelvic diaphragm is also the floor of the abdominal cavity, which contains the stomach, small and large intestines, liver, bladder, and kidneys. It lifts up and helps shape these vital organs.

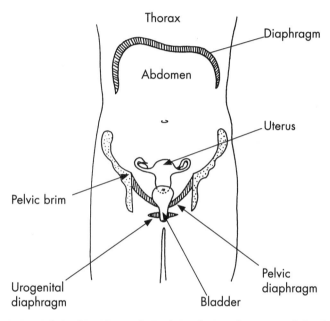

Fig. 1.2. Deep breathing issues from the pelvic and urogenital diaphragms.

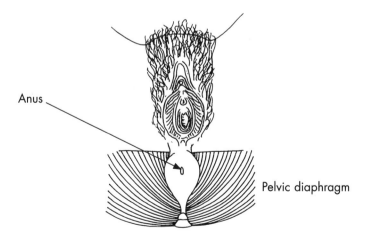

Fig. 1.3. Pelvic diaphragm

The Urogenital Diaphragm

At the perineum, the point midway between the anus and vagina, below the pelvic diaphragm, is another muscular diaphragm called the urogenital diaphragm. This is penetrated by the urethra, and on its underside it is attached the shaft of the clitoris (fig. 1.4).

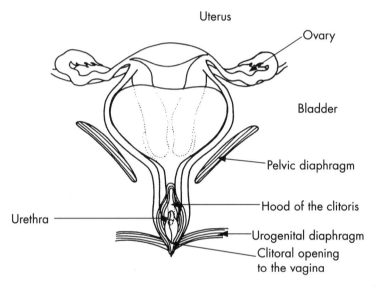

Fig. 1.4. Urogenital diaphragm

These two diaphragms seal and hold the life force, or chi, to prevent its escape through the lower openings in the body. When the openings that pass through these diaphragms are tightly sealed, chi pressure will be increased in the abdomen. When chi pressure strengthens, it will invigorate the vital organs, helping to improve the flow of chi and blood.

The Sacral and Cranial Pumps Move Chi Up the Spine

Contained and protected within your spinal column and skull is the very "heart" of your nervous system (fig. 1.5a). Cushioning it is the cerebrospinal fluid (*cerebro* for "the head" and *spinal* for "the vertebrae"). This fluid, as described by the Taoists long ago, is circulated by two "pumps." One is located in the sacrum and is called the sacral pump. The other is in the region

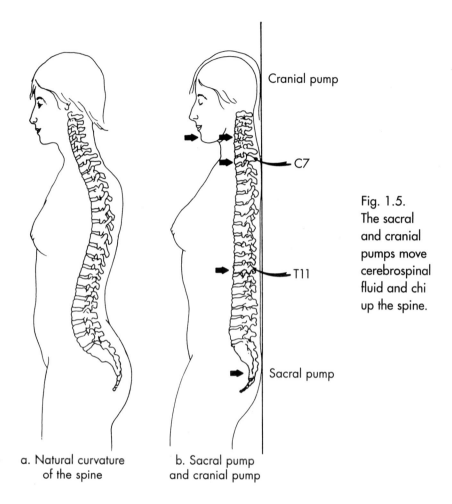

Cranial pump

C7

T11

Sacral pump

Fig. 1.5.
The sacral
and cranial
pumps move
cerebrospinal
fluid and chi
up the spine.

a. Natural curvature
of the spine

b. Sacral pump
and cranial pump

of your upper neck and head and is known as the cranial pump (fig. 1.5b). Many people who have activated these pumps have reported the sensation of a "big bubble" of energy traveling up their spine during Ovarian Breathing.

The Sacral Pump

Taoists regard the sacrum, which contains the sacral pump, as a point at which the sexual energy coming up from the ovaries and perineum can be held and then transformed as it is given an upward push. It can be compared with a way station that refines the energy of the ovaries, or Ching Chi, as it circulates in the body. If the opening of the sacrum to the spinal column (the sacral hiatus) is blocked, the life force cannot enter and flow up to the higher center.

The Cranial Pump

The Taoists have long regarded the cranium of the skull as a major pump for the circulation of energy from the lower centers to the higher centers. Medical research has recently confirmed that minute movements of the joints of the eight cranial bones occur during breathing. Cranial movement is responsible for the production and function of the cerebrospinal fluid surrounding the brain and spinal cord, and this is necessary for normal nerve and energy patterns in the body. Strengthening the cranial joints can increase energy and alleviate symptoms such as headaches, sinus problems, visual disturbances, and neck problems.

During Ovarian Breathing, we use the mind and a slight tensing of the neck and jaw to help activate the sacral and cranial pumps.

Perineum Power

Taoists regard the perineum region as the lowest diaphragm, one that functions like a pump. The perineum region is known as the seat of yin (cold) energy and is closely connected to the organs and glands (fig. 1.6). The Chinese term for perineum, Hui Yin, means the collection point of all yin energy, or the lowest abdominal energy collection point. It is also known as the Gate of Death and Life. This point lies between the two main gates. The front gate, or sexual organs gate, is the big life-force opening. Here the life force can easily leak out and deplete the organs' function. The walls of the vagina are tight during youth and after a refreshing sleep, but they

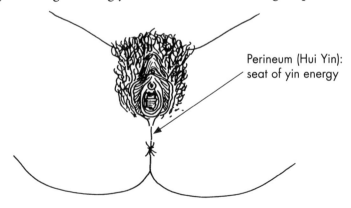

Perineum (Hui Yin): seat of yin energy

Fig. 1.6. The perineum

become looser as we age or when fatigued. The walls of the vagina, housing the PC muscle, must be strong in order to permit the life-force energy to flow and increase their strength. The second gate, the back gate, is the anus.

Control of the Chi Muscle influences the pumping action. As Ovarian Breathing floods this region with energy, the perineum, vagina, and anus begin to tighten almost immediately. In the Universal Tao practices, especially in Iron Shirt Chi Kung, the perineum's power to tighten, close, and draw the life force back up the spine is an important factor (refer to *Iron Shirt Chi Kung,* Destiny Books, 2006, for the complete Iron Shirt practice).

The Five Sections of the Anus

The anus is divided into five sections: middle, front, back, left, and right, which are closely linked with the chi of the organs and glands (fig. 1.7). When the anus is not sealed or closed tight, we can easily lose the nutrition needed for our life force and sexual energy through "a river of no return." By contracting and pulling up the various sections of the anus, energy is directed upward to the organs.

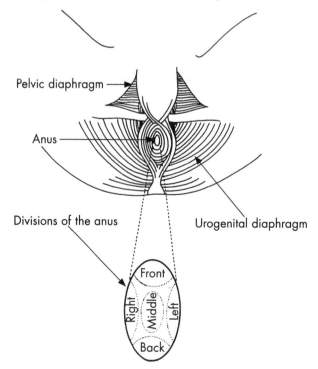

Pelvic diaphragm

Anus

Divisions of the anus

Urogenital diaphragm

Fig. 1.7. The anus is divided into five regions.

Right   Middle   Left

Front

Back

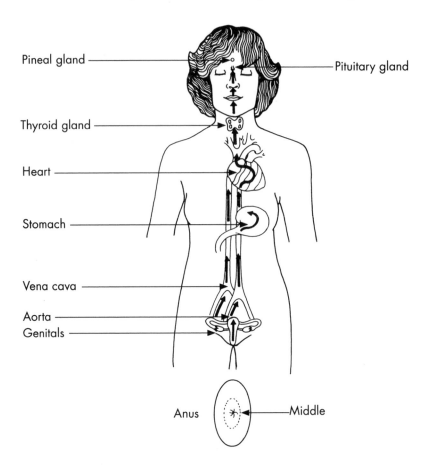

Pineal gland

Pituitary gland

Thyroid gland

Heart

Stomach

Vena cava

Aorta

Genitals

Anus — Middle

Fig. 1.8. Pulling up the middle part of the anus

Middle Part

The chi in the middle of the anus is connected with the following organs and glands: the vagina and uterus, aorta and vena cava, stomach, heart, thyroid, parathyroid, pituitary and pineal glands, and the top of the head (fig. 1.8).

Front Part

The chi in the front of the anus is connected with the following organs and glands: the bladder, cervix, small intestine, stomach, thymus and thyroid glands, and the front part of the brain (fig. 1.9).

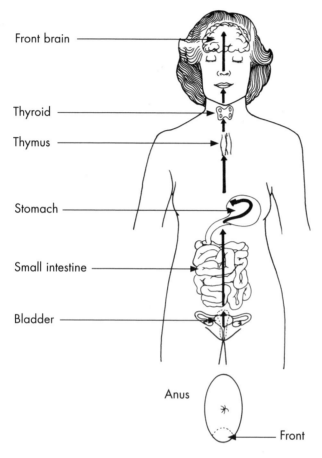

Front brain

Thyroid

Thymus

Stomach

Small intestine

Bladder

Anus

Front

Fig. 1.9. Pulling up the front part of the anus

Back Part

The chi in the back part of the anus is connected with the organ and gland energies of the sacrum, lower lumbar spine, twelve thoracic vertebrae, seven cervical vertebrae, and the cerebellum (small brain) (see fig. 1.10 on page 18).

Left Part

The chi in the left part of the anus is connected with the organ and energies of the left ovary, large intestine, left kidney, left adrenal gland, spleen, left lung, and the left hemisphere of the brain (see fig. 1.11 on page 18).

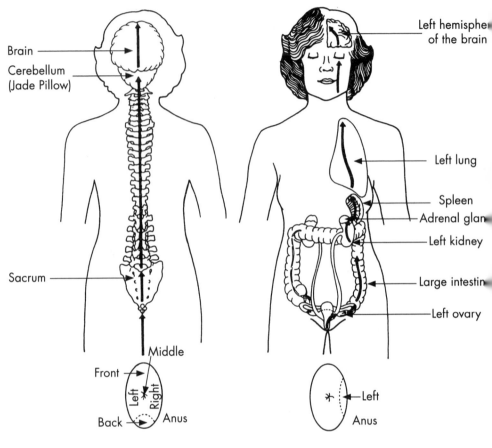

Fig. 1.10. Pulling up the
back part of the anus

Fig. 1.11. Pulling up the
left part of the anus

Right Part

The chi in the right part of the anus is connected with the organ and
gland energies of the right ovary, large intestine, right kidney, right adrenal gland, liver, gallbladder, right lung, and the right hemisphere of the
brain (fig. 1.12).

Once you are well trained in controlling the Chi Muscle, you can
easily guide the sexual healing energy to the particular organs or glands
that you need to heal, or guide the energy to help your partner during

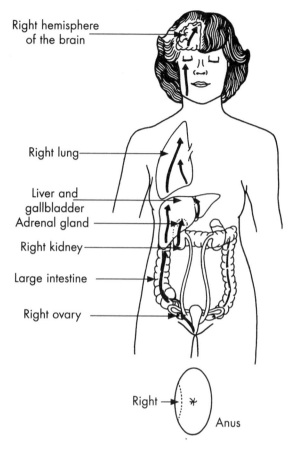

Right hemisphere
of the brain

Right lung

Liver and
gallbladder

Adrenal gland

Right kidney

Large intestine

Right ovary

Right →

Anus

Fig. 1.12. Pulling up the
right part of the anus

lovemaking. As you begin working with these exercises, remember that a contraction of the vagina is a contraction of the PC muscle, which initiates the contraction of the entire Chi Muscle group. Since the anus belongs to the area known as the perineum, we can say that "to contract and pull up the anus" is "to contract and pull up the perineum." Therefore the contractions of the Chi Muscle used in Ovarian Breathing are often expressed as "to contract and pull up the perineum."

OVERVIEW OF THE
OVARIAN BREATHING EXERCISE

The Ovarian Breathing exercise involves a gentle contraction of the Chi Muscle, as delicate as the closing petals of a flower and so minimal that anything less would have no effect at all. After bringing your awareness to both ovaries, you will gather energy in the area known as the Ovarian Palace, which you will learn to locate when we discuss the steps of the Ovarian Breathing exercise in detail. From the Ovarian Palace, you will move the energy through the uterus to the perineum. From there, you will guide it up your back to the brain, and then, using your tongue as a switch, you will guide it down to your navel, where it can be stored.

We have noted that the energy of the ovaries is regarded as hot energy. As such, it can be stored in the heart center or navel center. Some people store too much energy in the heart and find that it causes heartburn and difficulty breathing. This means there is excess energy that is not circulating sufficiently. Therefore, in the early stages of your practice, we advise you to store the sexual energy in the navel. As your practice continues, you can store it in the heart to increase love, joy, and compassion.

Postures

There are three postures in which to practice Ovarian Breathing: sitting, standing, and lying. It is best to begin practicing in a standing or seated posture and try other postures only later on, when you are more adept.

Sitting Posture

For simplicity and comfort, sit on a chair (fig. 1.13). Sitting lends ease to a practice that favors relaxation and good concentration.

Sit on the edge of a chair with both the legs and buttocks supporting your weight. Do not put all the weight on the sitz bones because in time this can create sciatic nerve pain. The vagina and perineum should not be constricted but should be covered with comfortable underwear or loose clothing to protect them from any draft. As a helpful technique used since ancient times to help the chi activate easily, you can place a hard, round object, perhaps a ball, in such a way that it presses directly on your vagina and clitoris during practice, or you can sit on the heel of one foot, pressing it tightly against the clitoris. If you already practice the Microcosmic Orbit circulation, you should be adept at directing energy upward and can omit this step.

Raise the tongue to the roof of the mouth: this is essential in circulating the chi and completing the loop between the front and back channels of the Microcosmic Orbit (fig. 1.14). Plant your feet firmly on the floor. Your back should be quite straight at the waist, but slightly round at the shoulders and neck. This very minor forward curvature of the upper back tends to relax the chest, and helps the power flow through the neck, chest, and abdomen. Keep the chin slightly tucked in. Military posture, with shoulders thrown back and head held high, tends to lodge power in the upper body and prevent its circulation back down to lower centers.

A variation on the sitting position is to sit cross-legged, either in the lotus position or Native American style. We appreciate the esoteric virtues of the lotus position, but Chinese practice attributes serious disadvantages to this way of sitting. Some monks suffered severe sciatic nerve pain or were crippled by lengthy meditation in the lotus position. Also, turning

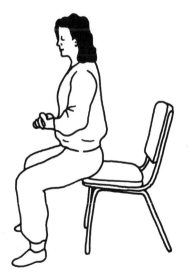

Fig. 1.13. Sitting posture

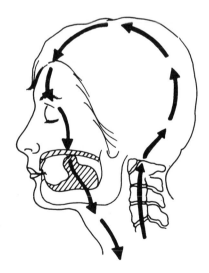

Fig. 1.14. The tongue touches the palate so the energy can flow down.

the soles of the feet away from the ground prevents you from directly drawing in the earth's yin power through the feet. When you are very good at controlling and directing the energy, you can sit in any position and still direct the energy as you wish. However, the human body is designed to absorb earth energy through the Kidney meridian (KD 1 point) and other meridians in the feet and filter it before passing it up to the coccyx and brain. Some people can develop problems if they absorb too much "raw" Earth Chi directly into their perineum and sacrum, as occurs in the lotus position. Eventually they can become allergic to this undigested energy and experience numerous unpleasant reactions. Nevertheless, those accustomed and devoted to the lotus position may use it, as long as they are comfortable and can apply their whole attention to the exercise. Few cross-legged positions afford the relaxation of the perineum provided by sitting on the edge of a chair.

Standing Posture

Standing is particularly favorable for Ovarian Breathing because it allows the sacrum and pelvis to relax. Standing up straight in a relaxed manner encourages good posture. Your hands should be at your sides and your feet shoulder-width apart. Discipline yourself to relax if you feel too tense, or the chi power may stick in the heart region and make you irritable.

The instructions on raising the tongue tip to the palate and maintaining correct posture given for the sitting posture apply also to this position.

Lying Posture

In the beginning, before you learn to control the energy, do not lie flat on your back when performing these exercises. In this position, the chest sits higher than the abdomen and receives too much energy. Nor should you lie on your left side. Both of these positions unduly stress the heart. The best way to practice Ovarian Breathing lying down is on your right side with a pillow beneath your head, your right leg extended, your left leg resting on your right thigh, and your right hand supporting your head.

Placing a pillow beneath your head should raise it about three or four inches, so the head sits squarely on the shoulders. Place the four fingers

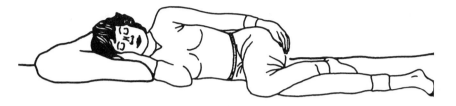

Fig. 1.15. Another way to practice Ovarian Breathing lying down

of your right hand immediately in front of your right ear, and place your thumb behind your ear, folding the ear slightly forward to keep it open. The ear must stay open to permit air to flow through the Eustachian tube and keep the pressures of the left and right ears balanced. This is important, because you can create a great deal of chi pressure during this practice. Rest your left hand on your outer left thigh. The right leg should be straight; the left leg, which rests on the right, should be slightly bent (fig. 1.15).

Lying on the right side can relieve the spine from stress. Lions often sleep in a similar position. Animals have a wise instinct, since this position frees the spinal column from the pressure of gravity, allowing it to assume its natural curvature. As mentioned previously, when you have mastered the energy well, you can lie on your back to practice, but make sure that the energy does not get stuck in the chest and heart. Do not lie on the left side.

Getting the Most from Your Practice

Before beginning, be sure your whole body is relaxed. If you are tense, do some stretching exercises or take a walk first in order to disperse tension. Allow all tension to flow out of you, as if you were in meditation.

In the Taoist practice sexual energy is the primary energy. If you only exercise the muscles and have no knowledge about life force and sexual energy, then the benefits are less. Use the mind alone to raise and lower the sexual energy.

With practice, you will learn to identify the hot Ching Chi stored in the area of the ovaries. Always start by breathing and collecting energy in the ovaries, until you get more familiar with the way the energy feels.

Unless otherwise specifically indicated, all breathing is to be done through the nose. Nasal breathing affords better control of the air inhaled. It filters and warms the air and supplies life force of a well-balanced quality.

All of your inhalations in the exercise should be short sips of air.

Ovarian Breathing Step by Step

In this section we will explain each step in the practice of Ovarian Breathing in great detail. In chapter 5, we have included a quick summary of the practice, to be used as a guideline only when you are more advanced.

Assume the Posture

Remember to wear loose pants or comfortable underwear to protect the vaginal opening from drafts and to avoid leakage of chi. Do not practice naked in a cold room, or you will lose a lot of chi. Of the three suggested positions, sitting or standing are preferable for this exercise.

> **Sitting:** Sit erect on the edge of your chair with your feet flat on the floor, approximately shoulder-width apart, palms on knees; chin tucked in; head held high (and, if desired, with a hard, round object placed so that it presses directly on your vagina and clitoris).
> **Standing:** Hands at sides; feet shoulder-width apart.

Bring Energy into the Ovarian Palace

1. Begin the exercise by locating the Ovarian Palace. Place both thumbs on the navel and use your index fingers to form a triangle. The place

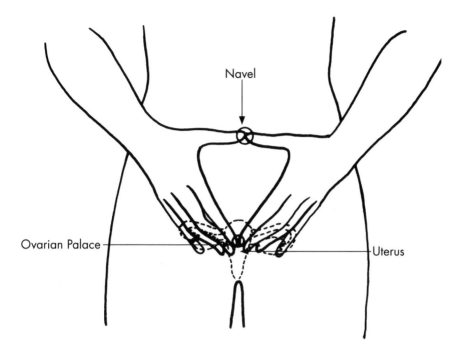

Fig. 1.16. Locating the ovaries and the Ovarian Palace

where the index fingers touch is the Ovarian Palace. Spread out your little fingers evenly: underneath the points where they rest are the ovaries (fig. 1.16).

2. Become aware of your ovaries as your fingers rest on them. Rub the ovaries until you feel them warming. Concentrate in order to produce more energy from the ovaries and eggs.

3. At the same time, use your mind to control the PC muscle to slightly close and open the vagina, as delicately as the petals of a flower. The energy may begin to manifest itself with such sensations as warmth, tightness, swelling, or tingling. Each woman can react differently to the energy.

4. When you start to feel something, inhale and bring the energy to the Ovarian Palace (where your index fingers touch). The gentle opening and closing of the vagina and the concentration of your mind gradually will enable you to collect and absorb the energy of the ovaries into the Ovarian Palace.

❂ *First Station: Perineum*

1. Concentrate on that warm feeling and mentally guide it from the Ovarian Palace to the front part of your perineum as you inhale a short sip of air. Pull the energy of the ovaries down to the perineum by contracting both the outer and inner lips of the vagina, pulling downward, and then contracting and pulling up the front of the anus (the perineum).

2. Be aware of the energy now flowing from the Ovarian Palace to the perineum. You might feel the route the energy follows from the uterus down through the cervical canal and along the back wall of the vagina down to the perineum, an action induced by setting your mind at the perineum to hold the energy there. The energy might make a detour to the shaft and glans of the clitoris before arriving at the perineum. In any case, you should feel the energy move from the Ovarian Palace to the perineum, whether or not you can feel the exact route it follows (fig. 1.17).

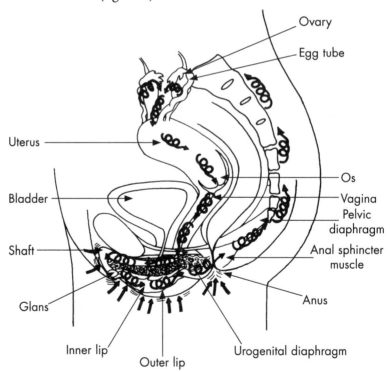

Fig. 1.17. Ovarian Breathing

3. Hold your breath, inhale in short sips, close the vagina tightly, and retain the energy of the ovaries at the front part of the perineum for a while. Exhale.

4. With each inhalation and exhalation counting as 1 repetition, repeat the process 9 times per session. Each time, return to the ovaries, and while you are there, inhale and exhale several times to build up more energy before you begin the process again.

Retaining the Sexual Energy at the Perineum Point

Retaining the Ching Chi at the perineum is very important, for if you release your attention, the warm energy will drop down and leak out of the vagina.

Think of drinking a full glass of water through a straw. You cannot draw all the water in one sip. You have to break the flow in order to breathe, and if you do not hold or retain the water that you already have in the straw, the water will flow out. In order to drink again you will have to begin drawing through the straw all over again. However, if you place your finger over the top of the straw while you breathe short sips of air, you can hold the water inside the straw.

By practicing, you will learn to use the power of the mind to hold the sexual energy at the perineum. Practice for several days, or until you are successful.

☯ Returning to the Ovarian Palace

As you strive to reach each energy transformation point in Ovarian Breathing, you must begin each time by returning to the Ovarian Palace to collect the energy of the ovaries.

1. Practice Ovarian Breathing by opening and closing the vagina slightly in order to collect the energy in the Ovarian Palace.

2. Once you feel that you have collected enough energy, repeat the process of bringing energy to the perineum. Each time, inhale a little sip of air and close the vagina with minimal movement of the Chi Muscle. At the same time you close the vagina, pull slightly downward toward the perineum, and then contract and pull up the front part of the perineum. Hold your breath, inhale in short sips, close the vagina tightly, and use your mind to create an awareness of the perineum point, thereby drawing the energy of the ovaries to this point. Retain the energy at the front part of the perineum. Exhale.

3. Upon exhalation, rest for a while, mentally guiding and feeling the Ching Chi as it travels from the Ovarian Palace down to the vagina, clitoris, and perineum, while maintaining your awareness of the perineum point and continuing to hold energy there.

4. Practice to this point for 1 to 2 weeks, or until you can definitely feel the energy at the ovaries, the Ovarian Palace, and the perineum. You will experience a sensation of energy traveling down to the vagina and a strong feeling as the energy moves gradually to the clitoris.

❷ Second Station: Sacrum, First Energy Transformation Point

Along with the ability to hold sexual energy, the sacrum also helps transform it into the first stage of life-force energy.

O Guide Energy to the Sacrum

1. Guide the ovaries' warm energy down from the Ovarian Palace to the perineum and up to the sacrum by first inhaling a short sip of air, slightly contracting and closing the vagina's outer and inner lips, pulling downward toward the perineum, and then contracting and pulling up the front part of the perineum.

2. Pause for a while, holding your breath; then inhale in short sips, close the vagina tightly, and retain the energy of the ovaries at the front part of the perineum. Be aware of the Ching Chi as it flows to this point.

3. Exhale and return to the ovaries, maintaining a part of your awareness at the perineum to retain the energy that you have brought there. Practice Ovarian Breathing by opening and closing the vagina slightly and collect the energy in the Ovarian Palace.

4. Once you feel that enough ovaries' energy has been collected, inhale and close the vagina, pulling downward toward the perineum, and then contract and pull the front part of the perineum upward to bring energy to this area. Rest briefly and be aware of the energy that travels from the ovaries down to the vagina, clitoris, and perineum.

5. Inhale slightly. Now pull up the middle part of the perineum, and at the same time pull up the back part of the perineum toward the coccyx at the very bottom of your spine.

O Activate the Sacral Pump

1. Slightly arch your lower back outward, tilting the sacrum downward to bring the energy to this point. As you pull the ovarian energy up the front, middle, and back parts of the perineum to the coccyx and then to the sacrum, hold the sacrum down to help activate the sacral pump (fig. 1.18). This action will be further accentuated if you gently tighten the back of your neck and skull bones. In the beginning, use a wall as a guide by pushing the sacrum against the wall, exerting force on it.

2. Hold the energy at the sacrum for a while, and then exhale, but continue to focus your attention on this point.

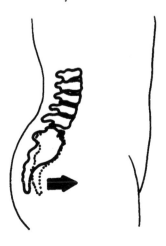

Fig. 1.18. Activating the sacral pump involves tilting the sacrum down without moving the hip bones.

O Open the Sacral Hiatus

The hiatus opening of the sacrum is an indentation in the bone of the sacrum, located a little higher than the tip of your spine. Once opened, this is the place through which you will draw your warm ovarian energy into the spine (fig. 1.19). This is usually a little difficult, because ovarian energy is denser than regular chi and has to be pumped through. Some people experience pain, a tingling sensation, or "pins and needles" when this energy enters the hiatus. If this happens to you, do not be upset. If you are having trouble, you can help pass the energy through the hiatus by gently massaging the area with a silk cloth from time to time.

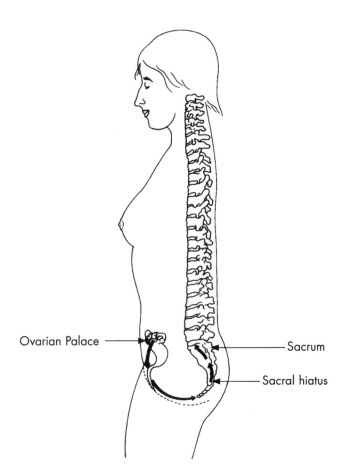

Fig. 1.19. Guiding energy through the sacral hiatus and
up the sacrum

O Rest in Order to Feel the Energy Move Unassisted

1. Now let your sacrum and neck relax back to their normal positions. As they relax you will feel the energy move by itself, assisted by the activation of both the sacral and cranial pumps. At the same time continue Ovarian Breathing.
2. Bring the energy up to the sacrum again and hold it there until you can feel the hiatus at the sacrum open and the energy gradually move up. You will actually feel the warm energy move up a little at a time.
3. Practice 9 times, then rest. The resting period is very important. Often, while you are resting, the energy will rise up through the point you were focusing on. If you can, still your mind and use it to guide the energy along the pathway you were working on, and then rest your mind and let the energy move by itself. You will find that the energy then automatically flows through that pathway.

O An Exercise to Help Open the Sacrum

If you have trouble feeling the energy at the sacrum, the following exercise can be helpful in opening the sacrum. The sacrum and the hips are three separate pieces of bone, which eventually become fused because we do not exercise them (fig. 1.20).

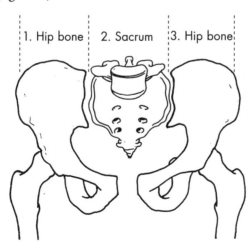

Fig. 1.20. The sacrum and the hip bones are
three separate pieces of bone.

1. Try rocking your sacrum back and forth and then hold the hips stationary, moving the sacrum only. Use both hands to hold the hips, and try to rock the sacrum. In the beginning it is difficult to do, but after a while you will gradually separate the hips from the sacrum.
2. You can also ask a friend to hold your sacrum with one hand with his other hand on your hip in order to let you know if it is the hip or the sacrum that you are moving.
3. Then hold still and observe the effect of the sacral pump working.

The Sacrum Helps Transform Raw Sexual Energy into Life-Force Energy

The Taoist masters discovered that the sacrum has the ability to transform sexual energy into a life-force energy that is more readily accepted by the organs and glands. Therefore, the practitioner must be aware of the state of the energy entering the middle part of the body. Some people practice by pulling up only the middle part of the perineum, causing the raw ovarian energy to shoot up the middle part of the body and become stuck in the organs and glands. Unaccustomed to handling this kind of raw sexual energy, the organs and glands may suffer from disorders such as indigestion, overheating (especially the liver), pain in the kidneys and back, and worst of all, heart congestion. These and other symptoms have come to be known as "Kundalini syndrome," and they occur when a person is not open enough to channel the raw sexual energy before it enters the vital organs.

This phenomenon is mentioned in the books *Kundalini— Psychosis or Transcendence?* by Lee Sannella, M.D., and *Stalking the Wild Pendulum* by Itzhak Bentov. These books contain many examples of people who suffered from the inability to control the rising energy. The energy they held in their hearts or in their heads was too raw or too hot for those organs, and they experienced allergic reactions to that energy. However, the symptoms disappeared once they learned about and felt the connection of the tongue to the roof of the mouth during the Microcosmic Orbit meditation. This connection allows the energy flowing up the spine through the major stations to transform into life-force energy and flow down to the navel. Many never know how to escape the problem of too much raw sexual energy rising up because they never learn how to bring the energy to the proper channels to circulate it back down.

Once you have practiced Ovarian Breathing and have felt the sexual energy circulate and become transformed, your organs will begin to adapt to and be able to withstand the raw sexual energy of the ovaries. This energy can then be directly transformed without problems arising.

✪ Third Station: T11, Sexual Energy Transformation Point

If you have managed to bring the energy up through the sacrum, spend the next week drawing the energy of the ovaries to T11 in your mid-back, opposite your solar plexus. T11 (the eleventh thoracic vertebra) also has the ability to transform the sexual energy into life-force energy. In Taoist practice we regard T11 as the energy center of the adrenal glands. The adrenal glands sit atop your kidneys and can act as a mini pump. When you arch the T11 point you create a vacuum in this area that pushes the energy up higher.

O Collect Energy in the Ovarian Palace

1. In the same manner as above, start with collecting the energy of the ovaries in the Ovarian Palace by opening and closing the vagina with a minimal movement of the Chi Muscle.
2. Inhale with a short sip and close the vagina slightly, pulling the energy downward toward the perineum. Then contract and pull up the front part of the perineum and pause for a while, holding your breath and retaining the energy at this point. Be aware of the Ching Chi that you have brought there.

3. Inhale in short sips, close the vagina tightly, and concentrate on retaining the energy of the ovaries at the front part of the perineum.

4. Exhale and return to the ovaries, but maintain a part of your awareness at the perineum to retain the energy that you have brought there. Continue to practice Ovarian Breathing, opening and closing the vagina slightly and collecting the energy in the Ovarian Palace.

O Draw Energy to T11

1. Once you feel that you have collected enough ovarian energy, inhale using a short sip and close the vagina by pulling downward, pulling the energy down to the perineum. Then contract and pull the front part of the perineum upward to bring energy to this area. Rest for a minute or two and be aware of the energy that travels from the ovaries down to the vagina, clitoris, and perineum.

2. Inhale a short sip and pull up the middle and back part of the perineum toward the coccyx to bring the energy to the sacrum. Slightly tilt the sacrum outward, as if you were pushing the sacrum to the wall. Pause for a while and feel the sacral pump activate.

3. Inhale a short sip again without exhaling, and tilt your spine outward against the imaginary wall to straighten T11. This will create an upward pumping action, which will pull the energy of the ovaries up to T11 (fig. 1.21).

4. Retain the energy at this point until the area feels full and until you feel the energy continue to open T11 and move up by itself. When you feel uncomfortable, exhale and regulate your breath.

O Flex the T11 Point to Help Activate the Pumps

1. As previously noted, ovarian energy is denser than chi. To accommodate it, flex the part of your back housing T11 in and out, thereby straightening and loosening the spine at this point for freer passage of the warm energy. Then allow your sacrum, T11, and neck to relax back to their normal positions. This action will help to activate the sacral and cranial pumps, as well as another mini pump located at

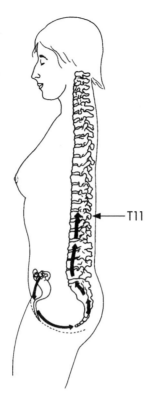

Fig. 1.21. Guiding energy up to T11

the adrenal glands, a little at a time. If you have trouble feeling this, return again to the Ovarian Palace and repeat the process.

2. Practice 9 times, then exhale and relax every part of the body. Concentrate on T11 and feel the energy flow up to this point.

❂ Fourth Station: C7, Sexual Energy Transformation Point

Your next stopping point is at cervical 7, or C7, located at the point of your spine at the base of your neck. You can feel it as the vertebra that sticks out when you bend your head down. This point controls the energy provided to the hands and neck, and is the connecting point providing power to the scapulae and spinal cord. This point also has the ability to transform sexual energy into life-force energy.

O Collect Energy in the Ovarian Palace

1. In the same manner as above, start with collecting the energy of the ovaries in the Ovarian Palace by opening and closing the vagina with a minimal movement of the Chi Muscle.
2. Inhale with a short sip and close the vagina slightly, pulling the energy downward toward the perineum. Then contract and pull up the front part of the perineum and pause for a while, holding your breath and retaining the energy at this point. Be aware of the Ching Chi that you have brought there.
3. Inhale in short sips, close the vagina tightly, and concentrate on retaining the energy of the ovaries at the front part of the perineum.
4. Exhale and return to the ovaries, but maintain a part of your awareness at the perineum to retain the energy that you have brought there. Continue to practice Ovarian Breathing by opening and closing the vagina slightly and collecting the energy in the Ovarian Palace.

O Draw Energy to C7

1. Once you feel that enough ovarian energy has been collected, inhale a short sip of air and close the vagina, pulling the energy of the ovaries downward toward the perineum, and then pull the front part of the perineum upward to bring energy to this area. Rest for a while and be aware of the energy that travels from the ovaries down to the vagina, clitoris, and perineum.
2. Inhale a short sip and contract the middle and back part of the perineum, and then pull the energy up to the sacrum, T11, and C7. When you reach C7, push slightly from the sternum to the back, and feel the push of C7 and both shoulders as they activate to draw the energy up (fig. 1.22). This action will activate the thymus gland to increase the upward pulling power. Hold the energy at this point as comfortably as you can. As you practice, you will find that gradually you are able to hold your breath longer and increase your capacity to intake air.

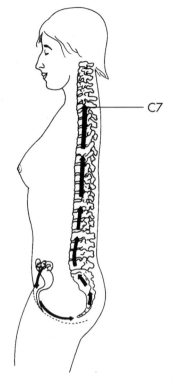

Fig. 1.22. Guiding energy up to C7

3. Exhale, and then let your sacrum, T11, and neck relax, returning to their normal positions. Concentrate on C7. This action will help to activate all three pumps (sacral, adrenal, and cranial) a little at a time. If you have trouble feeling this action, return to the Ovarian Palace and repeat the process.

4. Practice 9 times. Remember that you must return to the source of energy in order to bring it to the higher center.

☸ Fifth Station: Jade Pillow, Mini-Storage and Transformation Point

Your next stopping place is your Jade Pillow. This is located at the back of your head between cervical 1, or C1, and the base of the skull. This point also serves as a small storage and transformation point for sexual energy.

O Collect Energy in the Ovarian Palace

1. In the same manner as above, start with collecting the energy of the ovaries in the Ovarian Palace by opening and closing the vagina with a minimal movement of the Chi Muscle.

2. Inhale with a short sip and close the vagina slightly, pulling the energy downward toward the perineum. Then contract and pull up the front part of the perineum and pause for a while, holding your breath and retaining the energy at this point. Be aware of the Ching Chi that you have brought there.

3. Inhale in short sips, close the vagina tightly, and concentrate on retaining the energy of the ovaries at the front part of the perineum.

4. Exhale and return to the ovaries, but maintain a part of your awareness at the perineum to retain the energy that you have brought there. Continue to practice Ovarian Breathing by opening and closing the vagina slightly and collecting the energy in the Ovarian Palace.

O Draw Energy to the Jade Pillow

1. Once you feel that enough ovarian energy has been collected, inhale a short sip of air and close the vagina, pulling the energy of the ovaries downward toward the perineum, and then pull the front part of the perineum upward to bring energy to this area. Rest for a while and be aware of the energy that travels from the ovaries down to the vagina, clitoris, and perineum.

2. Inhale another short sip and bring the energy up to the sacrum, T11, and C7, then slightly push your chin down and pull it back, moving it toward the back of your neck at the base of your skull (fig. 1.23). Feel this push create a force that activates the cranial pump, which will help to pump the dense ovarian energy. Hold the energy at this point for a while, feeling it being stored and transformed.

3. Exhale, then permit your sacrum, T11, and neck to relax in their normal positions. This action will help to activate the adrenal, sacral, and cranial pumps again. Retain the energy at the base of the skull.

4. Repeat this entire process 9 times.

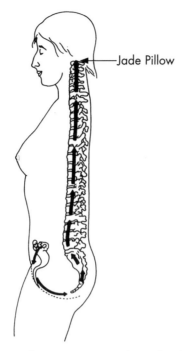

Fig. 1.23. Guiding energy up to the Jade Pillow

🌀 Sixth Station: Crown Point, Larger Storage Point for Sexual Energy

Your next stopping point, called the Crown point or Pai Hui, is located at the midpoint or crown of your head and is the center that houses the pineal gland. This is a larger storage point for sexual energy.

O Collect Energy in the Ovarian Palace

1. Practice in the same manner, only this time fill the "straw" to the top. Collect the energy of the ovaries in the Ovarian Palace by opening and closing the vagina with a minimal movement of the Chi Muscle.

2. Inhale with a short sip and close the vagina slightly, pulling the energy downward toward the perineum. Then contract and pull up the front part of the perineum and pause for a while, holding your breath and retaining the energy at this point. Be aware of the Ching Chi that you have brought there.

3. Inhale in short sips, close the vagina tightly, and concentrate on retaining the energy of the ovaries at the front part of the perineum.

4. Exhale and return to the ovaries, but maintain a part of your awareness at the perineum to retain the energy that you have brought there. Continue to practice Ovarian Breathing by opening and closing the vagina slightly and collecting the energy in the Ovarian Palace.

O Draw Energy to the Crown Point

1. Once you feel that enough ovarian energy has been collected, inhale a short sip and close the vagina by pulling downward to bring the energy of the ovaries to the perineum, and then contract and pull up the front part of the perineum to bring energy to this area. Rest for a while and be aware of the energy that travels from the ovaries down to the vagina, clitoris, and perineum.

2. Inhale and tilt the sacrum and T11 to the back in order to straighten the spinal curve out a little bit and thereby help activate the lower (sacral) pump. At the same time push the sternum in toward the back, tuck your chin in a little, and squeeze the back of your skull: this will activate the upper (cranial) pump. Continue pulling up to the point at the top, the center of the head (fig. 1.24).

3. As you continue to inhale, bring the energy down to the perineum, up to the sacrum, T11, C7, Jade Pillow, and then turn your eyes and other senses upward to help guide the energy up to the Pai Hui, or Crown point, and the pineal gland.

O Rest and Use Your Mind to Guide Energy to the Brain

1. Once the energy has finally completed its course up into your head, use your eyes and other senses to help retain it in the brain, holding it at the top of your brain as comfortably as possible.

2. Exhale, then let your sacrum, T11, and neck relax, returning to their normal positions. This will help to activate the three pumps: sacral, adrenal, and cranial. Use your mind to guide the energy station-to-station up the spine to the top of the head. Fix your attention and

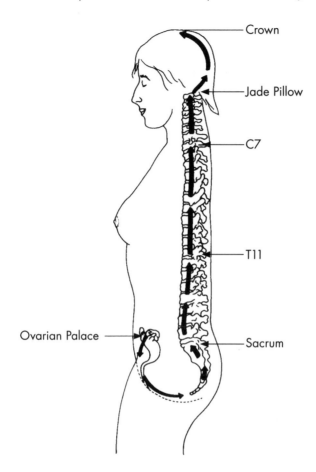

Crown

Jade Pillow

C7

T11

Ovarian Palace

Sacrum

Fig. 1.24. Guiding energy up to the Crown point

eyes at the Crown point. Remember it is the resting period that is the strongest in guiding the energy to the brain.

3. Repeat this process 9 times.

◉ Circulating Creative Sexual Energy in the Brain

As people age and use up much of their chi, they gradually drain themselves of brain energy and spinal fluids, drying them up and leaving a cavity. Ovarian Breathing transports creative sexual energy to refill this cavity and thereby revitalize the brain. Taoists regard sexual energy as similar to brain energy.

1. When you have finished practicing 9 times and can feel the sexual energy of the ovaries fill the brain, start to circulate the energy in the brain for 9, 18, or 36 counterclockwise revolutions. You should notice a very distinct feeling of spinning outward (fig. 1.25a).

2. When this circulation is completed, turn the energy back into the center of the brain for 9, 18, or 36 clockwise revolutions (fig. 1.25b). This should feel pleasant and energetic and will help to balance the left and right sides of the brain, revitalizing the brain to increase memory and facilitate clearer thinking.

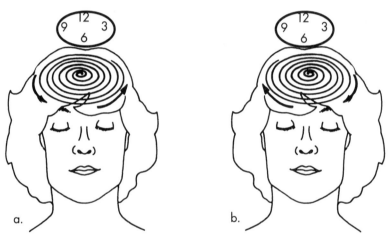

Fig. 1.25. Circulating energy at the Crown point

◯ Collect Sexual Energy at the Navel

It is very important to end your practice by storing the energy in the navel. An excess of energy in the head or the heart causes most of the ill effects of this practice. The navel can safely handle the increased energy generated by the ovaries.

1. Be sure the tongue is touching the palate (behind the front teeth will suffice) (see fig. 1.14 on page 21), so that the warm energy of the ovaries can flow down to the third eye, to the inside of your nose, and through the tongue from where it can travel down the throat to the heart center.

2. Retain the energy in the heart center for a while, filling it with energy until it feels open. Enjoy the feelings of love, joy, and peace; then bring the energy down to the solar plexus and to the navel. Collect the sexual energy at the navel, where it can be safety stored.

O Spiral the Energy around Your Navel Center

To collect the energy of the ovaries, concentrate on your navel area, about 1½ inches inside your body. Use your mind, eyes, and other senses to move the energy in and out, spiraling it around your navel. Do not spiral above the thoracic diaphragm or below the pubic bone.

1. Start by spiraling counterclockwise (outward) 36 times (fig. 1.26a).
2. Then reverse the direction of the spiral and bring it back to the navel, circling it clockwise 24 times (fig. 1.26b). Use your finger as a guide the first few times. The energy is now safely stored in your navel, available to you whenever and wherever your body needs it.

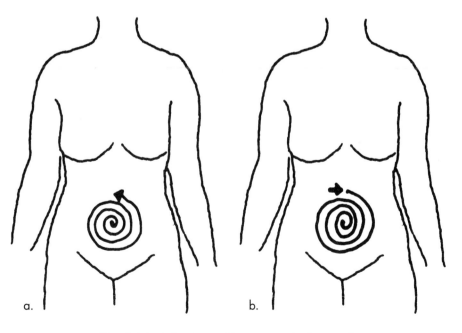

a.   b.

Fig. 1.26. Collecting smiling energy in the navel

Opening the Heart Center

Energy can also be stored in the heart center, which is a powerhouse for a woman. It is the seat of love, joy, and happiness, and is the center of rejuvenation, because it is the site of the thymus gland, which plays an essential role in the immune system. With this center open, you will experience all of these positive emotions and will be provided with abundant healing energy to heal yourself and others.

However, if the heart center is opened before you are ready, the Microcosmic Orbit will not be complete and the energy will not circulate property. The sexual energy can adhere to the heart, and the heat generated and congested there can cause problems such as uneasiness, shortness of breath, or pain in the chest. If you experience any of these problems, practice the healing sound of the heart as detailed in chapter 5. Lightly tap your chest and heart, and use your hands to brush your chest downward until you belch to release the trapped energy.

If you are a yang body type (meaning that your energy runs hotter than that of other people, perhaps manifesting in a hot temper), you should not start by storing the sexual energy in the heart. Instead, begin by storing it in the navel. Once the navel is filled, this is an indication that the channels are open enough to begin to store energy in the heart without problems.

☢ Collect and Spiral Energy in the Heart

To collect the energy of the ovaries in the heart, concentrate on your heart center located up 1 inch from the lower tip of the sternum, and about 1½ inches inside your body. It is approximately 3 inches in dimension. Use your mind, eyes, and other senses to move the energy in and out, spiraling it around your heart center. Do not spiral below the pubic bone.

1. Start by spiraling around your heart center counterclockwise (outward) 36 times (fig. 1.27a).
2. Then reverse the direction of the spiral, returning the energy to the heart center, circling it 24 times (fig. 1.27b). Use your finger as a guide for the first few times. The energy is now safely stored in your heart center, available whenever and wherever your body needs it.

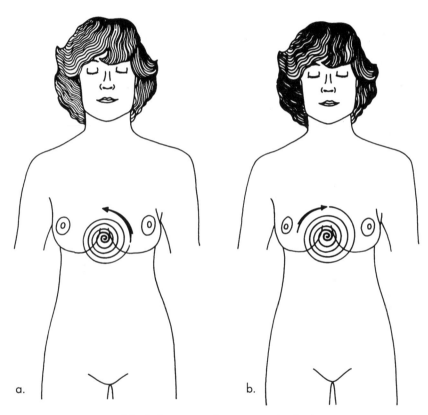

Fig. 1.27. Collecting smiling energy in the heart

🌀 Bringing Energy to the Brain with One Action

In the beginning of your practice, it is best to simply travel from station to station until you feel that the back channel, or Governor Channel, is more open.

1. Once you have mastered the process, you can practice the Ovarian Breathing exercise and the energy will travel up to the brain in one sweet drawing-up of the "straw," with a single, clean inhalation and one contraction of the vagina. Eventually all you will need is your concentration on both your ovaries and the crown of your head to mentally move the sexual energy from the ovaries all the way up to the brain in one step.

2. Exhale, then inhale and bring the energy up again.

3. Practice this a few times, but since the ovarian energy is warm, be sure to put your tongue up to your palate and bring the energy down to the navel.

One session of Ovarian Breathing should take about 10 minutes. When practiced 4 to 7 times a week, women have noticed changes in their menstrual cycles, such as less bleeding, decreased cramping, and a reduction in breast pain. With continued practice, menstruation may cease. The energy conserved in this manner becomes part of the vital energy of the body, increasing the amount of energy available for transformation into a higher form. There is also historical evidence that women who practice Ovarian Breathing have very healthy, well-balanced children, once they decide to have children.

Some perform Ovarian Breathing and then proceed directly to the Microcosmic Orbit meditation. The practice can be done any time and virtually anywhere, once you have achieved the direct pathway from the ovaries to the brain. When you find yourself with unstructured time—waiting in line, driving, sitting at your desk, watching television—carry out several series of contractions, or as many as you choose to fill the time available. The main consideration is that your back is properly straight, your chest relaxed, and your vagina protected from the breeze. You must also remember to touch your tongue to your palate after you practice 3 or 4 times.

The Effects of Ovarian Energy

Now that you are in touch with your ovarian energy, notice how it feels. Some women say the energy moving up their spine feels wide, thick like honey, and slow. Most women who perceive the temperature at all say it feels warm. Some women experience it as cool at first, but after practicing for a while, notice that it becomes warm. Some experience sensations in their genitals or on their thighs, usually describing them as warm to hot. Many women describe the energy as warmer, wider, heavier, or thicker than the organ chi that is circulated in the Microcosmic Orbit. This is because ovarian energy is heavier and denser than chi.

It is not unusual for the energy to feel cold when there is a lot of healing going on, such as with women who have menstrual problems. The sensations may vary over time. What is most important to understand is that if the energy feels warm, it must be circulated back down to the navel and not left up in the head.

Take your time to really feel the warmth when you practice. Do not rush it, and always maintain the action of the pumps as you breathe in and out. Use a more mental than physical pull when you do the exercise. Let the warm feeling be your guide. Always remember to bring the energy down to the navel after a few breaths, since the navel is roomy and a safe place to store this warm vital energy.

Ovarian Breathing tones the pelvic diaphragm. The whole lower abdomen is deeply massaged each time the pelvic diaphragm flexes. Life force flows into the region on periodic waves of breath, which stimulate the glands and vital organs.

Ovarian Breathing also has tremendous implications for women's control over their reproductive systems. There is too little evidence to come to any conclusions about the effectiveness or reversibility of this method when used for birth control. However some women are experimenting with this method, trusting that it will be reversible just by stopping the practice for a couple of months.

These women feel justified in using themselves as their own laboratories, since the method is gentle and appears to be under control, especially in the context of so many women who, out of desperation to control their reproductive systems, have already accepted the wholesale experimentation of dangerous birth control methods, by supposedly trustworthy institutions, such as IUDs, DES, morning-after pills, sequential birth control pills, and forced sterilization.

OVERVIEW OF THE OVARIAN COMPRESSION EXERCISE

Many of the benefits of Ovarian Breathing are magnified when performed in conjunction with the Ovarian Compression exercise. This exercise will help you consciously direct energy into and out of the pelvic region and pack chi into the ovaries and vagina. As an expanding sensation fills the genital area, sexual energy increases, eventually reaching into higher centers of the body through the Microcosmic Orbit, as it is needed. This practice is particularly important to use after the Sexual Energy Massage or Chi Weight Lifting to replenish the energy extracted from the ovaries.

By packing the chi into the ovaries and the vagina, you warm up the sexual region so that you can be more sexually active, more easily aroused, and more easily brought to orgasm. When the sexual region lacks chi, it gets cold and is difficult to arouse. This can be likened to attempting to boil ice water, as opposed to water at room temperature: it takes much more heat to bring ice water to the boiling point. By warming the ovaries, Ovarian Compression will warm your heart as well. It helps you calm down when sexually overexcited. It also reduces mental problems, strengthens the ovaries and the cervix, and increases the power of the vaginal muscles.

In this exercise you will inhale a fairly large amount of air into the throat and swallow it. Swallowing drives the air down to the solar plexus. From the solar plexus, you roll the air down into the pelvic region then drive it down both sides of the vagina to be compressed there. This is accomplished by contracting the abdominal muscles downward in a slow wave (fig. 1.28). The vagina will seem to expand, you will feel a flush of heat, and after a short time the power driven into the vagina will flow up your spine to your head, which will also become very warm. Remember to keep your tongue up on your palate when compressing the air.

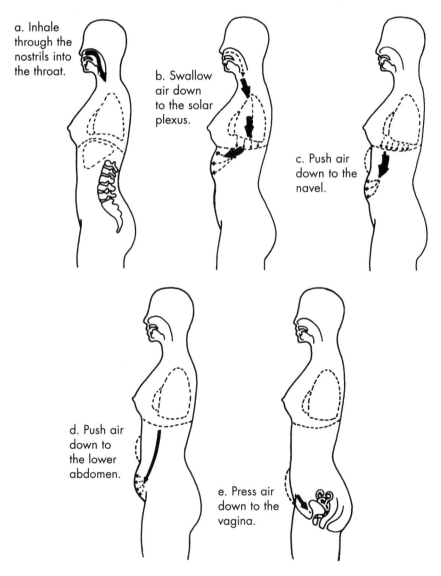

a. Inhale through the nostrils into the throat.

b. Swallow air down to the solar plexus.

c. Push air down to the navel.

d. Push air down to the lower abdomen.

e. Press air down to the vagina.

Fig. 1.28. Ovarian Compression

Ovarian Compression Step by Step

The three postures recommended for Ovarian Breathing also apply to Ovarian Compression. Of the three suggested positions, sitting or standing are preferable for this exercise. Sit on the edge of your chair with your feet flat on the floor, about shoulder-width apart. Feel your feet support a part of your weight; do not place all of your weight on the sitz bones. Wear loose clothing so that it will be easy to compact the chi.

1. Inhale through the nostrils into the throat. From there, swallow the air down to the solar plexus, midway between your heart and your navel. Do not stop at the heart center. Imagine the air as a ball of chi.

2. Feel the energy of each breath culminate at a point behind the solar plexus. From the solar plexus, roll the "chi ball" down to the navel, then into the pelvis, and spread it out to both sides of the ovaries. To accomplish this, contract the abdominal muscles downward in a slow wave.

3. Feel the chi pressure drop around the ovaries, pack and compress the ovaries to energize them, and gradually pack the cervix. Squeeze the inner and outer lips of the vagina tightly, and keep on pushing into the vagina as if you were blowing up a balloon, until the vagina feels as if it is expanding.

4. Forcibly compress air into the ovaries for as long as you can. Once the air is driven into the ovaries, you will experience a flush of heat. Every single compression shoots tremendous energy into the vagina. Each compression should last a minimum of 30 to 40 seconds. Slowly work up to at least 1 minute. With compression that lasts an entire minute, the exercise will take full effect. The anal sphincter and perineum muscles must be squeezed tightly during this exercise to prevent leakage of energy.

5. Keep your tongue pressed against the roof of your mouth to maintain the flow of energy through the Microcosmic Orbit. Move it around to stimulate the saliva flow. Swallow deeply into the sexual center to enhance the compression. When you have finished the compression, exhale and

relax completely. Swallow the accumulated saliva before exhaling.

6. After complete exhalation, take a number of quick, short breaths by pulling your lower abdomen in and pushing it out (Energizer or Bellows Breathing) until you are able to breathe normally. Relax completely. Remember to breathe through the nose, and do not inhale unduly large quantities of air.

7. In the beginning perform 2 to 3 compressions, gradually increasing to 9. When you have grown stronger you may do 9 compressions in succession, and then rest by rotating your body from the waist. Begin a second series of 9 compressions. Keep the breathing between compressions short and shallow so you do not lodge power high in the body.

❂ Quick Energy Recharge

If you feel ill or out of sorts, several Ovarian Compressions will restore you to good form, as this exercise charges the whole body. Try the following sequence:

1. First practice one Ovarian Compression.
2. Next, rotate the waist with the arms at shoulder level.
3. Rest for a moment and repeat.

Practice Ovarian Breathing and Ovarian Compression twice a day for approximately 15 minutes in the morning and 15 minutes in the evening. Regular practice of these breathing techniques will yield many benefits in addition to those already mentioned, such as a decrease in insomnia and nervousness and an improvement in overall energy.

The exercises should start to take effect within 3 days after you begin practicing. The ovaries will feel warm and may itch or feel somewhat tingly, an indication that the ovaries are receiving unusually high amounts of vital force. These signs will occur only if you are doing the exercise properly. A month or two of exercise will produce substantial increases in strength and well-being.

VENTING EXERCISES FOR
HIGH BLOOD PRESSURE

After practicing Ovarian Compression for two to six weeks, some women with high blood pressure notice a large flow of chi to the head. They feel tension in the head because the blood has followed the upward flow of the vital power. This is not unlike a mild symptom of "Kundalini syndrome," in which freed energy races about the body out of control.

If you suffer from high blood pressure and have not practiced meditation to open the Microcosmic Orbit, which distributes the energy evenly throughout the circuits of the body, you can vent excess pressure by meditating on two points. These are the Ming Men, or Door of Life, located on the spine directly opposite the navel (between the lumbar vertebrae 2 and 3), and the Yung Chuan, the kidney point (KD 1), located on the soles of your feet. The Ming Men is regarded as a very important safety point, as well as the strengthening point of the kidneys.

If blood flows too strongly to the head during or after Ovarian Compression, vent the power by practicing the Ming Men and Yung Chuan exercises right after compression. Imbalanced force will flow down the body through these two points.

 Using the Ming Men Point to
Vent Chi Pressure

1. To find the Ming Men, place a string around your waist like a belt. Make sure it is perfectly horizontal, and place it across your navel. The Ming Men lies where the string meets the spine. When you bend over backward from the waist, the point feels like a hole in the spine (fig. 1.29).
2. Meditate on the Ming Men point by smiling to the area and guiding excess chi in the head down to this point. Here it may be cleaned, balanced, and safely recirculated.
3. You can use your hands to help induce the downward flow of chi: envision the right hand sending out energy like a pitcher and the left hand receiving it like a catcher.

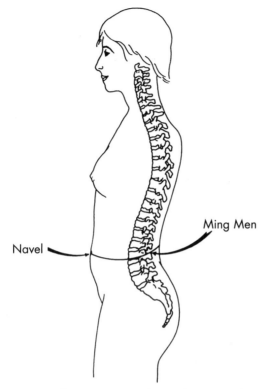

Fig. 1.29. The Ming Men is located opposite the navel
between the second and third lumbar vertebrae.

 ## Using the Yung Chuan Point to Vent Chi Pressure

The Yung Chuan point is the yin energy entry point. The Taoists regard the soles of the feet as the roots of the body, and the root is important as the foundation for the work of the spirit body.

1. Locate the Yung Chuan points on the soles of your feet (see fig. 1.30 on page 54).
2. Once you have found the points on both feet, tape onto them spiny little balls such as prickly chestnuts or plane tree seed pods. Place both soles on the ground and press firmly on the spiny balls while concentrating on the Kidney 1 point (also known as the Bubbling Spring).

3. Help to guide the energy down to the soles by placing your left palm on the sacrum, and your right palm on the top of your head. After a short time of practice you will feel the power flow to the Ming Men. Direct it down through the spine and backs of the legs to the Yung Chuan. Press down on the balls of the feet so that you feel the soles very distinctly. In severe cases it may take a month or two to get the power into the Ming Men and bring it down to the Yung Chuan.

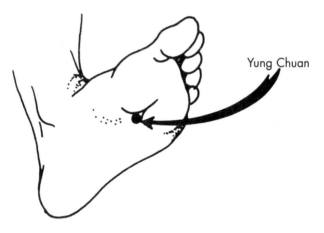

Fig. 1.30. Yung Chuan (KD 1) Point

After practicing these exercises, many students open the Microcosmic Orbit so that their energy flows in a continuous circuit, and there is no need to bring the energy down through the back to the soles. You can also bring it down the front of the body through the heart and navel, down to the perineum, and down to the backs of the knees to the soles. This alone has often ended high blood pressure.

POWER LOCK EXERCISE FOR WOMEN

The Power Lock should be practiced before and after the Sexual Energy Massage (presented in chapter 2) to assist in the upward draw of released energy and sexual hormones from the perineum to the crown. Air is inhaled through the nose in nine sips as the vagina, perineum, and anus are simultaneously contracted to draw Ching Chi upward. In conjunction with

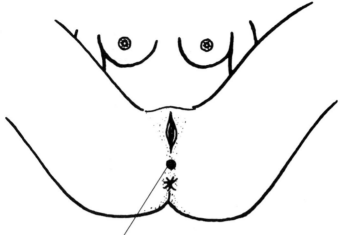

Fig. 1.31. Perineum and the point where pressure should be applied

these contractions, the three middle fingers of either hand are applied to a point at the back of the perineum, near the anus (fig. 1.31).

How to Apply the Pressure

Fingernails should be cut short and filed. Using either hand, combine the three middle fingers into a triangle. Immediately after each inhalation, press the three fingertips on the point in front of the anus to lock the Ching Chi into its upward journey, preventing its return to the perineum. Release the fingertips as you sip in more air and then reapply them as each breath is held. Press the point only for as long as you hold each breath and muscular contraction, then release. Do not apply the fingers as you inhale because you will block the energy from rising. Remember that the fingers help to push the energy upward. (You may forego using the fingers if it causes discomfort.)

Warning: Before you begin drawing Ching Chi up to the higher centers, remember that you should never leave hot sexual energy in the head for long periods of time. Always draw it down to the navel through the Functional Channel (front) of the Microcosmic Orbit at the end of your practice. There is an old Chinese saying: "Don't cook your brain." When in doubt about the hot or cold status of your energy, store it in the navel.

Activating the Pumps at the Five Stations

The pressure at the perineum helps to guide the rising energy up to five stations: the sacrum, T11, C7, base of the skull, and the crown (fig. 1.32). Each of the five stations has a "pump" to move energy, but the sacral and cranial pumps require the most concentration to become activated. Activating the pumps is done in sets using nine muscular contractions of the lower trunk simultaneously with nine sips of air to draw the energy up to each point from the perineum. The exercise then starts again at the perineum after each station has been completed, although the energy is actually held at the previous station.

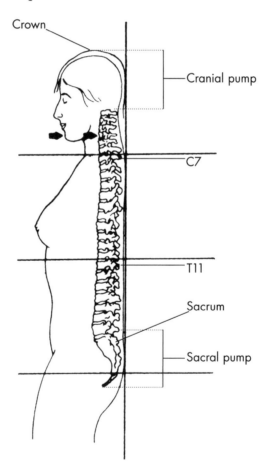

Fig. 1.32. Sacral pump and cranial pump

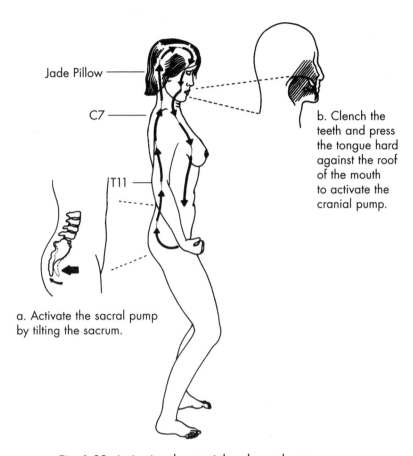

Jade Pillow

C7

T11

b. Clench the teeth and press the tongue hard against the roof of the mouth to activate the cranial pump.

a. Activate the sacral pump by tilting the sacrum.

Fig. 1.33. Activating the cranial and sacral pumps

To direct the energy up the spine, tilt the sacrum slightly and clench the buttocks as you contract the anus and perineum (fig. 1.33a). As the sacral pump is activated, it creates a vacuum in the urogenital diaphragm, which draws the Ching Chi up from the sexual center. The cranial pump is activated by first pressing the flat part of the tongue up to the roof of the mouth as the tip of the tongue presses the lower jaw behind the teeth (fig. 1.33b). Your teeth should be slightly clenched as you pull in the chin toward the back of the head. Take in 10 percent of your lung capacity with each sip of air through your nose as you pull up the sexual center, apply pressure with the three fingers, and contract the individual sections of the perineum region. Simultaneously push up your tongue, pull in your eyes, and look up to your crown.

Note: Remember never to contract the chest muscles. This can cause energy to congest around the area of the heart.

Sequence

Begin with Ovarian Breathing, slightly contracting the vagina to accumulate Ching Chi in the Ovarian Palace. Then use a short inhalation to draw the energy through each successive point leading up to the first station. Remember to apply the fingers as you hold each sip of air. First inhale and contract the perineum. Then inhale again as you contract the anus. With the next sip of air, pull up the back part of the anus as you draw the energy up to the sacrum. After covering these points, use several sets of nine contractions to push the energy into the sacrum. This entire sequence is repeated for each subsequent station.

As Ching Chi expands in the sexual center, use one sip of air with each contraction to draw it up through the aforementioned points. At least one set of nine contractions should be used for each station that was previously opened. Then emphasize each new station with several sets of nine contractions. Although a week or two may be required to open each station completely, you can practice using all of the stations, concentrating more on the difficult points. Exhale after the ninth sip of air, and release the tension as you repeat the process.

Power Lock Practice Step by Step

⚙ Station One—the Sacrum

1. Begin with Ovarian Breathing, slightly contracting the vagina to accumulate Ching Chi in the Ovarian Palace.
2. When you feel the Ching Chi expanding, inhale a sip of air and contract the perineum, drawing sexual energy into the perineum. Use your fingers to press on the point each time you inhale and contract, releasing them briefly before each subsequent contraction.

3. Inhale, contract the anus, and draw the energy from the perineum up to the anus.

4. Inhale, contract, and draw the energy up to the back part of the anus.

5. Inhale, and tilt the sacrum as you clench the buttocks to activate the sacral pump. Draw the energy up to the sacrum.

6. Use 9 contractions with 9 sips of air to draw Ching Chi from the sexual center to the sacrum (fig. 1.34).

7. Hold the energy at the sacrum as you exhale and return your attention to the sexual center.

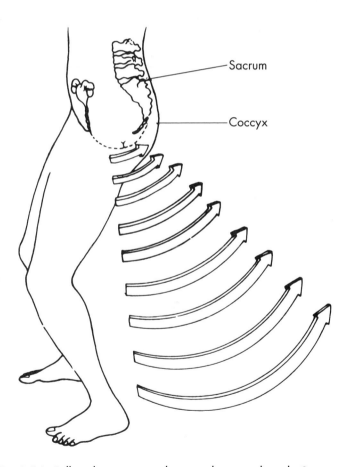

Fig. 1.34. Collect the energy at the sexual center; then do 9 contractions
to draw the energy to the sacrum.

✪ Station Two—the T11 Point

Repeat the previous steps, drawing the energy up through the sacrum until you reach the T11 point.

1. Use 9 contractions with 9 sips of air to draw the Ching Chi from the sexual center to T11 on the spine. (Activate the T11 pump by pushing the spine outward at that point.)
2. Hold the energy there as you exhale and return your attention to the sexual center.

✪ Station Three—the C7 Point

Repeat the previous steps, drawing the energy up through T11 until you reach the C7 point.

1. Use 9 contractions with 9 sips of air to draw Ching Chi from the sexual center to the C7 point. (Push the C7 out, and pull back the chin slightly to help activate the C7 pump.)
2. Hold the energy there as you exhale and return your attention to the sexual center.

✪ Station Four—the Base of the Skull

Repeat the previous steps, drawing the energy up through C7 until you reach the base of the skull.

1. Use 9 contractions with 9 sips of air to draw Ching Chi from the sexual center to the base of the skull as you activate the cranial pump. (Pull the chin back once again.)
2. Hold the energy there as you exhale and return your attention to the sexual center.

☯ Station Five—the Crown

Repeat the previous steps, drawing the energy up through the base of the skull until you reach the Crown point (fig. 1.35a).

1. Use 9 contractions with 9 sips of air to draw Ching Chi from the sexual center to the crown (see fig. 1.35b).
2. Exhale and rest as you spiral this energy 9 times outward from the crown, and then 9 times inward.
3. Finally, bring the energy down and store it in the navel.

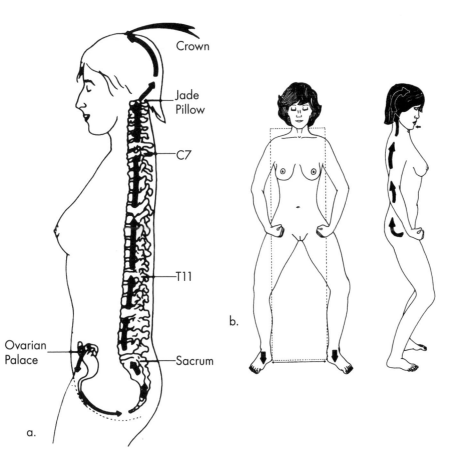

Fig. 1.35. Power Lock: guiding the energy up to the crown

❂ Completion of the Power Lock

Cover your navel with both palms, right hand over left. Collect and mentally spiral the energy outward from the navel 36 times counterclockwise, and then inward 24 times clockwise (fig. 1.36).

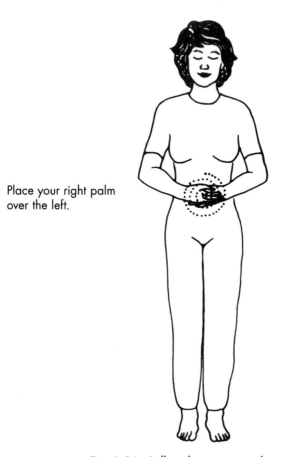

Place your right palm over the left.

Fig. 1.36. Collect the energy at the navel.

Sexual Energy Massage and Internal Egg Exercise

Taoists regard sexual energy as having creative and rejuvenating powers. They acknowledge its role in the conception of human life, but when procreation is not intended, they advocate other applications for Ching Chi. In the Healing Love practice, this energy is used to heal the internal organs and glands, increase the brain's capacity, and further open the channels of the Microcosmic Orbit. In the more advanced practice of the Sexual Energy Massage, it is also used to replenish and cultivate the blood-producing red marrow of the bones.

In the Internal Egg Exercise a stone egg is inserted into the vagina, which provides a marvelous way to strengthen and control the Chi Muscle. It is easier to practice control of this muscle with an egg in the vagina, because as the egg moves, you can distinctly feel the direction in which the Chi Muscle moves. Controlling this voluntary muscle means controlling the many involuntary muscles in this area as well. Also, as you master the use of this muscle of the vagina and perineum, you will simultaneously tone up the lower abdomen.

SEXUAL ENERGY MASSAGE

The Sexual Energy Massage is a beginner's equivalent to Chi Weight Lifting, which requires much more experience and qualified instruction. The massage draws sexual energy and hormones into the body and promotes a healthy flow of blood and chi within the sexual center. It also brings more internal energy into the genitals and increases the production of Ching Chi. Using these techniques, women often alleviate the problems associated with menstruation.

The Sexual Energy Massage often causes enough stimulation to require the Healing Love techniques to avoid sexual arousal. If arousal occurs, draw the activated sexual energy into the Microcosmic Orbit. The Power Lock should be used before the Sexual Energy Massage to prepare for the procedures, and afterward to draw Ching Chi up through the stations of the Microcosmic Orbit. At least two to three sets are recommended at both times.

An extremely important preparation for the Sexual Energy Massage techniques is the Cloth Massage of the sexual center, which stimulates the energy and prepares the sexual organs for the role at hand. The perineum and sacrum are also massaged since they are powerful stimulators of life-force energy.

 ## Cloth Massage

A silk cloth is used to massage the genital area, the perineum, the coccyx, and the sacrum. Silk works well because it develops considerable static energy when rubbed. This is important for the stimulation of chi. First, the silk cloth is applied to activate Ching Chi. The Sexual Energy Massage then releases the Ching Chi to be assimilated into the body. While massaging with the cloth, women should feel the breasts enlarge slightly as the vagina becomes moist with secretions. Using the cloth should help you feel the chi routes open as they are stimulated.

The Cloth Massage of the sexual center, perineum, and sacrum should also be repeated after the Sexual Energy Massage or Chi Weight Lifting, to replenish the circulation of blood and chi in the sexual center.

1. Hold the cloth using the three middle fingers of either hand. Apply the cloth directly to the sexual center (including entire mons and labial area) in clockwise and counterclockwise motions for 36 rotations in each direction (fig. 2.1). Massage the vaginal muscles, pressing in on the sides of the groin.

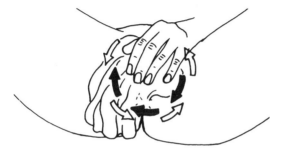

Fig. 2.1. Cloth Massage

2. Locate the perineum, and use the cloth to massage it clockwise 36 times and then counterclockwise 36 times.
3. Apply the cloth to the coccyx and massage its tip, gradually applying more pressure to activate the sacral pump. Massage clockwise and then counterclockwise 36 times. Move up to the sacrum and massage it clockwise, then counterclockwise 36 times (fig. 2.2).

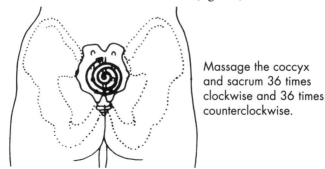

Massage the coccyx and sacrum 36 times clockwise and 36 times counterclockwise.

Fig. 2.2. Massaging the sacrum

Sexual Energy Massage

The Sexual Energy Massage should always be preceded by the Cloth Massage of the sexual center, perineum, and sacrum. The Sexual Energy Massage can be followed by the Internal Egg Exercise, which is useful in all sexual activities and is a prerequisite for Chi Weight Lifting.

Breast Massage

Massaging the breasts activates the sexual energy of the ovaries, which subsequently activates the energy of the glands and the organs. It is also possible to prevent lumps from forming within the breasts, or to dissolve them, by using this practice. You should find that this practice greatly enhances your health and sexuality.

1. Begin in a seated position, either naked or wearing loose pants. You should feel a firm pressure against the vagina. To achieve this, sit up against a hard object, or place a rolled up towel between your legs. If you are naked, use a sanitary cover for protection.
2. Pull up the middle and back parts of the anus, drawing the chi up through the spinal cord (fig. 2.3). Then pull up the left and right sides of the anus, and bring chi directly up to the left and right nipples.
3. Warm the hands by rubbing them together as you inhale, and press the tongue against the roof of the mouth. Place the second joint of the middle finger of each hand directly on the nipple of its respective breast. Cup the outside of the breasts with your palms.

Massaging the Glands with Accumulated Chi

As you do the following exercise, combine the chi stimulated in the breasts with the additional energy of each successive gland or organ, drawing it back up to the breasts as the energy of each is activated. Return to the breasts after each of the following steps. Think of the breasts as melting pots for the combined ingredients of chi from the organs and glands.

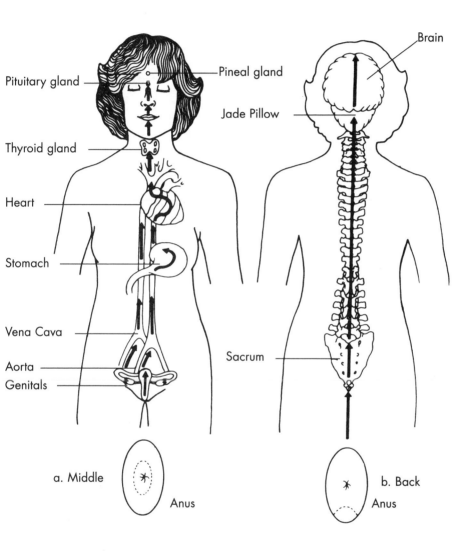

Fig. 2.3. Pull up the middle and back parts of the anus.

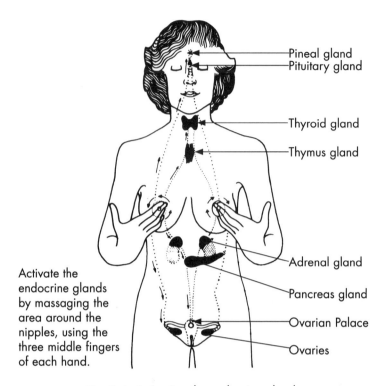

Pineal gland
Pituitary gland

Thyroid gland

Thymus gland

Adrenal gland

Pancreas gland

Ovarian Palace

Ovaries

Activate the endocrine glands by massaging the area around the nipples, using the three middle fingers of each hand.

Fig. 2.4. Activating the endocrine glands

1. Use the three middle fingers on each breast to circle outward from the nipples and then inward again. Move your right hand clockwise, and your left hand counterclockwise, then reverse. Direct the chi accumulated in the breasts to the glands (fig. 2.4).

2. When the clitoris is energized, the sexual energy surges to the head and activates the pineal gland at the crown. Return your attention to the breasts.

3. Continue massaging as you move your attention to the pituitary gland, behind the "third eye," or mid-eyebrow point. You may feel pressure in the head as the energy descends to the pituitary gland. Return your attention to the breasts.

4. Draw the activated energy down to the thyroid and parathyroid glands. Feel the expansion of these two glands as they become activated. Return both your attention and the chi to the breasts.

5. Continue to gently massage the breasts, and settle your attention on the thymus gland in order to activate its energy. Return your attention to the breasts with the combined chi.

6. Let the chi flow down to the pancreas to activate it. Return the combined chi to the breasts.

7. Activate the adrenal glands with the energy, and bring it up to the breasts to blend with all the energies of the other glands. This accumulation will help to activate the chi of the organs.

◉ Massaging the Organs with Accumulated Chi

1. Again, rub your palms together until they are hot, and cover your breasts with your hands. Feel the chi from the thymus and the breasts activate the energy of the lungs (fig. 2.5). Direct this chi back to the breasts.

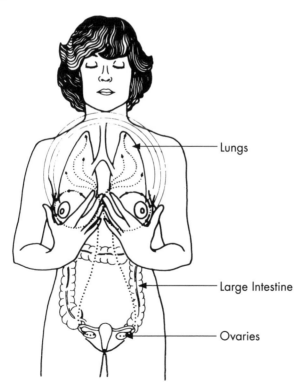

Fig. 2.5. Activating the chi of the lungs and large intestines

2. Activate the heart's energy with the accumulated chi, and direct this energy to the breasts.

3. Direct your attention to your spleen, and allow the accumulated chi to activate the spleen's energy (fig. 2.6). Feel the chi of the spleen, and direct it to the breasts.

4. Now direct the chi to the kidneys (fig. 2.7). Activate the energy of the kidneys, and direct it to the breasts.

5. Direct the chi to the liver, and activate its energy (fig. 2.8). Draw the liver's energy into the breasts.

6. Place your palms on your knees as you focus your attention upon your breasts. Experience the energy that has accumulated in them. Let the energy expand into the nipples as you feel a tingling warmth. Wait a few moments as the breast energy accumulates in the nipples, and

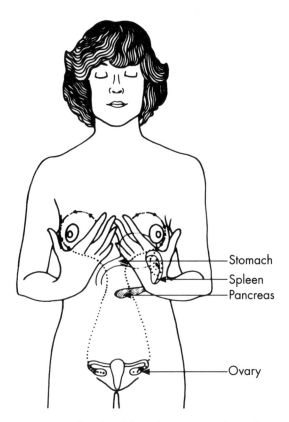

Fig. 2.6. Activating the chi of the spleen, stomach, and pancreas

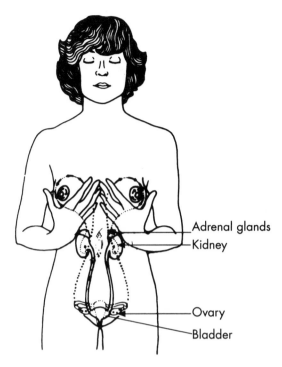

Fig. 2.7. Activating the chi of the kidneys, adrenal glands, and bladder

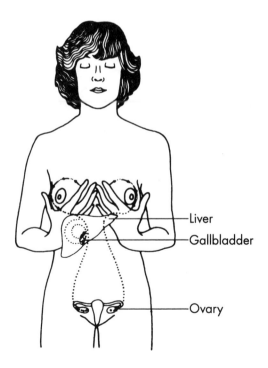

Fig. 2.8. Activating liver and gallbladder chi

then let the energy flow directly down into the ovaries. Pause, and feel the accumulated energy in the ovaries.

7. Become aware of your breath and concentrate on the ovaries, breathing directly into them. Use your mind and a slight muscular contraction to move the lips of the vagina. Feel an increase in the pulsation of the vagina, and feel it open and close like the petals of a flower. When this energy becomes strong, let the vagina close in, and then draw the energy from both ovaries to merge in the Ovarian Palace, located 3 inches directly below the navel. Slightly squeeze in, tense the cervix, and concentrate the sexual energy at this point.

Incorporating Breast Self-Examination into Your Practice

Breast cancer is the leading cause of cancer death in women. If discovered early enough, it can be successfully treated. To protect yourself, we suggest that once a month, ideally after your menstrual period, you incorporate into your practice the simple technique of breast self-examination for early detection of breast cancer. Always feel thoroughly for any changes your breasts may have undergone since your last checkup. Stand in front of a mirror and examine their appearance. Is there any unusual dimpling or puckering of the skin, discoloration, ulceration, hardening, or lumpiness? Have the superficial blood vessels grown larger or increased in number? Has the size, shape, or contour of your breasts changed? Next, elevate your hands above your head and ask yourself the same questions.

While massaging your breasts, be sure to note any lumps, thickening, or changes in the texture of your breasts, and tell your doctor if you notice anything unusual. Don't overlook the tissue under your arms. Western health care practitioners recommend a yearly mammogram for women over the age of forty.

🔄 Massaging the Ovaries

After completing the breast massage, place each hand over its respective ovary at a hand's breadth below the navel on each side of the abdomen, and massage the ovaries 36 times in both directions as you did with the breasts (fig. 2.9). The chi that is now available for your practice is comprised of energy from the organs, the glands, and the sexual center.

The Sexual Energy Massage prepares the vagina for the practice of the Internal Egg exercise. Once you have sufficiently stimulated the breasts and the clitoris, the warm, moist vaginal secretions indicate that the body is ready for the egg to be inserted.

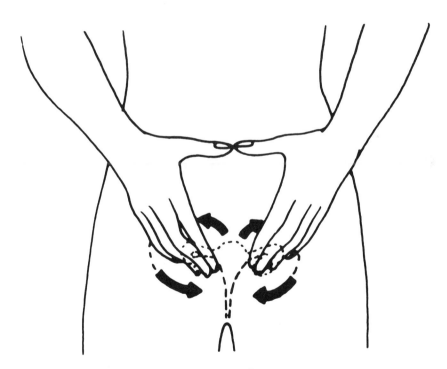

Fig. 2.9. Massage the ovaries,
circling 36 times in both directions.

OVERVIEW OF THE INTERNAL EGG EXERCISE

In ancient China the egg exercise was a closely guarded secret of the queen and concubines who aimed to please the king. Taoist women used it to strengthen the sexual region, thereby increasing both the Ching Chi and life-force energy that was available to them. This practice also helps the practitioner to develop internal strength and control over her sexuality. A stone egg is inserted into the vagina and then moved up and down the vaginal canal. This internal workout increases the strength of the lower abdomen and fosters the development of mastery over the Chi Muscle. It also aids in gaining control over many of the involuntary muscles in the same area. The egg exercise helps to improve spiritual as well as physical health, since these exercises provide more power to the Chi Muscle to lift the sexual energy inward and upward, where it can be transformed into higher spiritual energy.

Selection and Care of the Egg

Eggs made of jade or obsidian are recommended for this exercise. Jade eggs are preferred because they are sturdy, smooth, and nonporous. You may also find that jade eggs are far less expensive. Wooden eggs or any eggs with painted or chemical finishes should be avoided. The egg should be drilled to accommodate a string passed through its center for the advanced weight-lifting practice. Even if weights are not used, the string can help in removing the egg. Gem and mineral shops generally have a large selection of sizes and materials of eggs, as well as a range of prices. These eggs are also available through the Universal Healing Tao (contact information can be found at the end of this book).

The eggs range in size from that of a quail egg to a jumbo supermarket egg. You will need to decide what size looks as if it might feel comfortable in your vagina. Most women choose a medium-sized one, that is, an egg approximately one inch in diameter. The smaller the egg, the more work your muscles will have to do, because they will have to contract more strongly to cause any movement of the egg.

Cleanliness of the egg is extremely important. All eggs should be boiled prior to their first use. Also be sure to clean the egg thoroughly after each use, as mucous secretions on the egg are an ideal medium for bacterial growth. Jade eggs can be boiled daily, although washing may suffice. Boil the egg at least once a week for complete safety, and never let anyone else use your egg. Because some women may be unknowingly allergic to isopropyl or rubbing alcohol, avoid using them to clean the egg.

Caution in Practicing the Egg Exercises

The following suggestions should be kept in mind as you initiate your practice:

- Before practicing the egg exercises, you must first master Ovarian Breathing.
- Do not practice lying down.
- If you have a tight vagina, or if you are a beginner, use the egg with a string to eliminate any fears of the egg becoming stuck. Ultimately, you will learn how to expel the egg without the help of the string. If an egg without a string attached gets stuck, do not panic. Relax and allow the muscles to rest until you can gradually expel the egg.
- When the perineum grows stronger you may wish to advance to a double egg system.
- If the preliminary massage does not provide enough natural lubrication, lubricate the egg with a nontoxic oil or gel prior to its insertion. Be sure that the lubricant is not petroleum-based.
- Proper feminine hygiene is an absolute necessity for these practices. This exercise should not be attempted if you have a vaginal infection or if you are menstruating. Wait at least two days after your period is over before starting practice.
- The best time to practice the Sexual Energy Massage and the Internal Egg Exercise is in the morning, preferably after bathing.

Three Areas of Contraction

The egg is used as a guideline for contractions in three specific locations, as shown in figure 2.10.

1. The first is the front of the vaginal canal, within the external orifice.
2. The second is the middle of the canal between the first and third sections.
3. The third is directly beneath the cervix, near the end of the canal.

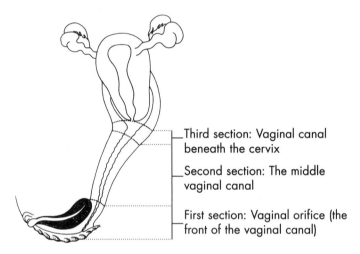

Fig. 2.10. Three sections of the vagina

Each section is contracted individually, beginning with the external orifice, then the middle canal, and then the anterior of the cervix, which is contracted before beginning once more at the orifice. The egg's use is unnecessary if you prefer to initiate the internal contractions without it. In that case the egg is only needed for Chi Weight Lifting. In contraction exercises without an egg, the Chi Muscle—which encompasses the anal, perineal, and pubococcygeus muscles—is used to contract the three sections of the vaginal canal. The egg exercise, used in conjunction with the Sexual Massage, creates more resistance within the canal. Chi Weight Lifting is the final stage of the practice in which maximum resistance can be attained.

Internal Egg Exercise

The importance of a preliminary Cloth Massage before practicing the Egg Exercise and Chi Weight Lifting cannot be overlooked. Its purpose is to stimulate hormone secretion from the breasts and ovaries.

1. Begin the massage by gently but firmly pushing the fatty tissue of the mound of each breast against the rib cage, moving two or three fingers of each hand in small circular movements. Start at the central nipple areas and work your way around and outward until each entire breast has been massaged. Both sides can be worked simultaneously if a long enough piece of cloth is used.
2. Insert the egg into the vagina, larger end first.
3. Once inserted, assume the standard Horse stance posture (feet shoulder-width apart and firmly grounded, ankles and knees bent, groin folded, spine and neck in alignment). Assume a clenched-fist position with your palms facing upward. It is from this basic rooting stance that each phase of the egg exercise is performed (fig. 2.11).
4. Isolate and contract the first section of the vaginal canal, the muscle groups responsible for closing the external vaginal orifice tightly. This will help keep the egg in the vaginal canal.

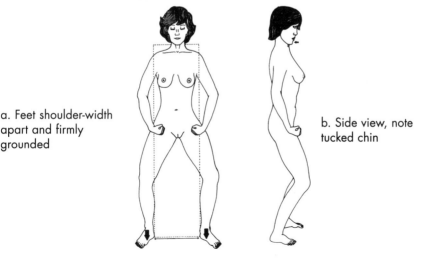

a. Feet shoulder-width apart and firmly grounded

b. Side view, note tucked chin

Fig. 2.11. Horse stance for the Internal Egg Exercise

5. As the egg is pushed into the vaginal canal, an internal sucking action is begun by contracting the three sections of the canal to move the egg in and out of each section. The sequence of contractions is as follows:

a. Inhale and contract the muscles immediately in front of your cervix while keeping the first set of muscles contracted (fig. 2.12).

b. Using the muscles in the middle of the vaginal canal, lightly squeeze the egg. Inhale and squeeze harder, then move the egg up and down. When you are out of breath, exhale and rest (fig. 2.13).

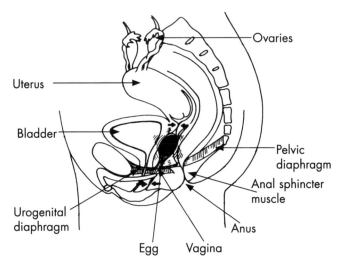

Fig. 2.12. Pushing the egg into the vaginal canal

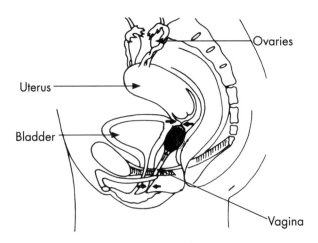

Fig. 2.13. Moving the egg up

c. Use the top set of muscles—those in front of the cervix—to move the egg left and right, then rest (fig. 2.14). Now use the bottom set of muscles (controlling the vaginal orifice) to move the egg left and right (fig. 2.15).

d. Use the top set of muscles, then the bottom set, to tilt the egg up and down. Combine all of the movements, then slide the egg up to touch the cervix and down to the vaginal orifice. Release.

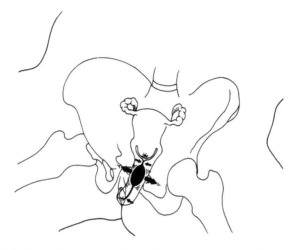

Fig. 2.14. Using the top set of muscles to move the egg left and right

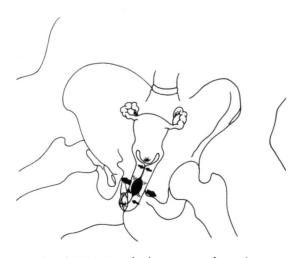

Fig. 2.15. Using the bottom set of muscles
to move the egg left and right

6. The speed of the motion should eventually be increased and maintained until you feel the need to rest. The rest period is important, as it is at this time that chi will start to accumulate in the area.

7. Take a deep breath and draw the accumulated energy into the Microcosmic Orbit.

8. You should remove the egg by contracting the vaginal muscles to expel it. At first, a squatting position may be necessary. Try elevating one leg on a short chair to facilitate the egg's removal. If you are using an egg with a string attached, removal should be very simple, although your internal capabilities should be allowed to develop without too much external help.

9. Massage the breasts and vaginal areas with a silk cloth after practicing the egg exercise (fig. 2.16).

10. Next, massage the perineum in a circular motion counterclockwise for 9, 18, or 36 times, and then clockwise for 9, 18, or 36 times. Massage the coccyx and sacrum in the same manner using a counterclockwise motion, and then reverse for the same number of repetitions.

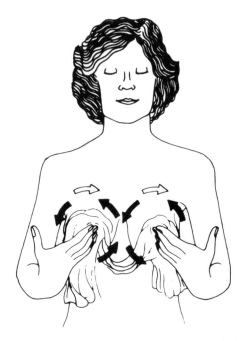

Fig. 2.16. Massage the breasts with the cloth.

This will enhance the action of the sacral pump and increase the upward flow of chi, transforming raw sexual energy into life-force energy.

11. Rest, then practice 2 or 3 of the Six Healing Sounds, particularly the lung and heart sounds. (See chapter 5 for instructions on practicing the Six Healing Sounds.) Also practice the Microcosmic Orbit meditation to circulate the tremendous energy you have generated throughout your body. Sit comfortably, concentrate on the navel, and use the mind to move the energy.

☸ Using the Egg during Ovarian Breathing

Once the Internal Egg Exercise is mastered, it can be combined with Ovarian Breathing. Each will enhance the practice of the other.

1. Prepare yourself with breast massage until you feel ready, and insert the egg into your vagina.

2. Align your body in the basic Horse stance described earlier.

3. Close the external vaginal orifice by isolating and contracting the individual muscle groups responsible for tightly closing the orifice.

4. Gather the energy from the ovaries and the breasts at the Ovarian Palace. Inhale slowly and deeply. Draw the sexual energy down through the uterus to the clitoris and hold it there.

5. Grip and move the egg. Contract and hold the lower, then the middle, and then the upper vaginal muscles, feeling your grip on the egg. Then push the egg deeply up into the vaginal canal. Move it up and down and feel the increasing sexual energy.

6. As you feel more energy gather at the vaginal canal, follow the procedures of Ovarian Breathing. (If necessary, please review the details of the practice of Ovarian Breathing in chapter 1.) Pull the energy to the front part of the perineum, to the sacrum, T11, C7, C1, Jade Pillow, and Crown point. Circulate the energy in the brain and bring it down the front channel to the third eye, tongue, throat, heart center, solar plexus, and navel. Collect the energy at the navel.

☯ *Two Eggs Technique*

You can upgrade the practice by using two eggs in the vagina at the same time, moving them up and down or in different directions, or banging them together to achieve a vibration that will stimulate the internal organs (fig. 2.17). Two eggs are more difficult to manage, like drawing a square and circle simultaneously using both hands. It is important to know how to manage one egg well first.

Once you are well trained and are master of your Chi Muscle, you can dispense with the eggs, and instead use your mind and the appropriate muscles to move the sexual energy as you wish.

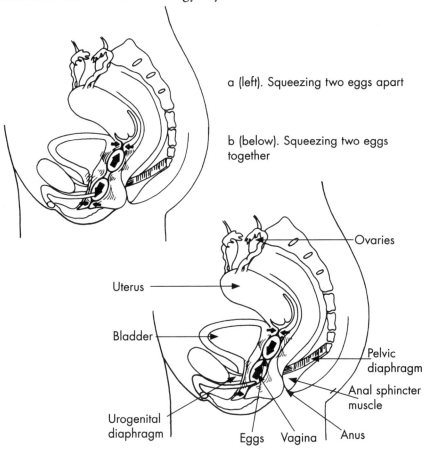

a (left). Squeezing two eggs apart

b (below). Squeezing two eggs together

Ovaries

Uterus

Bladder

Pelvic diaphragm

Anal sphincter muscle

Urogenital diaphragm

Eggs   Vagina   Anus

Fig. 2.17. Internal Egg Exercise using two eggs

Chi Weight Lifting

Chi Weight Lifting is included in this text solely for the documentation of its procedure to serve as a guide for instructors and trained students of the Universal Healing Tao. It is not intended for beginning students. Universal Healing Tao cannot and will not be held responsible for any reader of this book who attempts Chi Weight Lifting without first receiving qualified instruction.

The ancient Taoist masters discovered that the genitals were connected to the organs and glands in the area of the perineum called the Chi Muscle, which encompasses the anal, perineal, and pubococcygeus muscles (see fig. 3.1 on page 84). With this knowledge they developed the Healing Love techniques, using the Chi Muscle to create an upward flow of sexual energy into the higher centers of the body. They eventually learned to increase this chi flow by developing the fascia, the connective tissue around the organs and glands (see fig. 3.2 on page 84). In the Chi Weight Lifting practice for women the fascia is engaged by the organs and glands to lift weights attached to an egg held in the genitals. The beneficial aspects of strengthening the internal system through the fascia became an integral part of Bone Marrow Nei Kung.

Originally men accomplished Chi Weight Lifting by placing stones in a basket and hanging the basket from their groins. Today, male and female Taoists use light weights to draw a special formula of sexual energy from the genitals upward into the body. This sexual energy, or Ching Chi, is

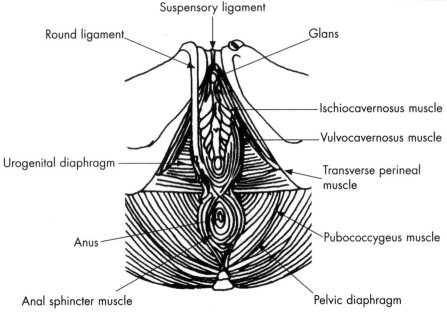

Fig. 3.1. Chi Muscle includes the urogenital diaphragm,
the pelvic diaphragm, the anal sphincter muscle,
and the pubococcygeus (PC) muscle.

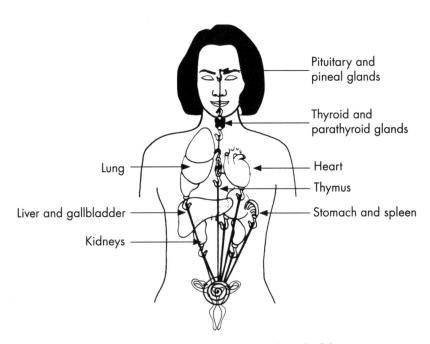

Fig. 3.2. Sexual organs are joined to all of the
organs, glands, tendons, and muscles.

combined with external energy and compressed into the skeletal structure through the methods described in this book. As sexual energy transforms into life-force energy, Chi Weight Lifting enhances the life force of those who practice it. The genitals are replenished by the rejuvenated organs and glands as the transformed energy returns through the Microcosmic Orbit.

In addition to Sexual Energy Massage and Chi Weight Lifting, Bone Marrow Nei Kung also includes the practices of Bone Breathing, Bone Compression, and Hitting with a bundle of wire rods or rattan sticks. Bone Breathing uses the power of the mind, along with deep, relaxed inhalations, to establish an inward flow of external energy through the fingertips and toes. This energy is used to complement previously stored sexual energy, which is released into the body through the Sexual Energy Massage or Chi Weight Lifting and then compressed into the bones using Bone Compression. The Hitting techniques are employed to detoxify the body, stimulate the lymphatic and nervous systems, and compress chi into the bones. A summary of the Bone Breathing and Bone Compression techniques is provided in chapter 5 of this book, while detailed instruction in Hitting can be found in chapter 4 of *Bone Marrow Nei Kung* (Destiny Books, 2006).

BENEFITS OF CHI WEIGHT LIFTING

In Chi Weight Lifting, an upward counterforce is created by the internal organs and glands to resist weight that is suspended from an egg held in the vaginal canal.

Strengthens the Fascial Network

The upward counterforce created by the organs is strengthened by the chi released from the sexual center as the internal system engages the fascia to pull up against the weight. The fascia, therefore, contributes greatly to the distribution of energy. It also serves as the connection between the sexual organs and the pelvic and urogenital diaphragms. When this connection is loose, the Chi Muscle and the diaphragms allow the organs to drop their weight onto the perineum, thereby reducing the chi pressure. When the connection is kept strong, the organs and glands are held in place and the chi pressure is maintained.

Creates Powerful Urogenital and Pelvic Diaphragms

The human body has many diaphragms holding the internal organs and glands in place, such as the thoracic, pelvic, and urogenital diaphragms. During Chi Weight Lifting these contribute greatly to the upward counterforce deployed against the downward pull of the weights anchored to the genitals (fig. 3.3). The pelvic and urogenital diaphragms, considered the floor of the organs, and the Chi Muscle are all strengthened by this practice, which helps to prevent any loss of energy through them. Their increased strength also helps to alleviate the protruding abdomen caused by organs stacking up on the pelvic area (fig. 3.4).

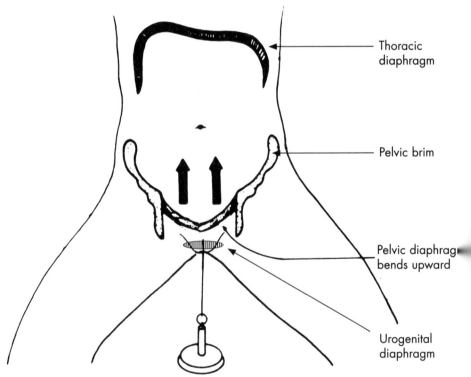

Thoracic diaphragm

Pelvic brim

Pelvic diaphragm bends upward

Urogenital diaphragm

Fig. 3.3. The pelvic and urogenital diaphragms provide counterforce to the weights.

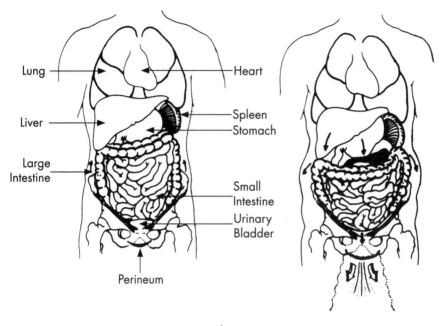

Fig. 3.4. The organs

Chi Weight Lifting is credited with many other benefits related to the improved functioning of the diaphragms, such as the lifting of dropped kidneys. Furthermore, the practice helps to seal the openings of the anus and vagina to prevent the leakage of chi. Taoists believe that this helps to redirect the spirit away from these openings as one prepares to finally leave the body. The upward flow of energy that is developed through Taoist practices will point toward the crown as the proper exit for the spirit to use at the end of life.

Delays the Aging Process

The release of sexual hormones stimulates the pituitary gland to prevent the production of an aging hormone. It has been proposed that one function of this gland may be to measure the growth of mutated reproductive cells. Scientific studies have found some evidence that the aging hormone is released when these mutations are allowed to increase beyond a certain level. Theoretically their growth should be impeded by a healthy reserve of sexual hormones. Otherwise, upon sensing the reduced presence of

Ching Chi within the body, the pituitary gland can cause a premature death by producing the aging hormone. It is therefore wise to maintain sexual energy and hormones through the Taoist practices.

Stimulates the Brain

The right side of the brain is also influenced by the sexual hormones to promote the healing and rejuvenation of the body. Since Ching Chi revitalizes the internal system and regenerates the bone marrow, hormonal stimulation of the brain greatly enhances these processes. This effect also serves Taoist spiritual work because practitioners find it to be an invigorating experience on all levels. The health of the body and the mind directly affects the spirit.

EQUIPMENT AND EXTERNAL PREPARATIONS FOR CHI WEIGHT LIFTING

Equipment

You will require a special jade or obsidian egg drilled lengthwise for the insertion of a string to hold the weight (see chapter 2). The egg is inserted into the vagina, large end first, with the string tied to the weight. Squatting may make it easier to insert the egg as the weight rests on the floor. The weight is then lifted and swung like a pendulum.

Women can begin Chi Weight Lifting with a ½-pound weight, gradually adding ½ pound at a time. Light weights are available, which can be tied directly onto the string. Or the string can be tied to the men's weight-lifting apparatus, first using it alone as a trial weight (fig. 3.5). The apparatus is made from an 8-inch length of 1-inch diameter galvanized pipe with a ¼-inch hole drilled through the pipe ½ inch from either end. At one end, a heavy ring 1½ inches in diameter is attached. Any of several different types of clamps (used in standard barbell sets) may be used on the opposite end of the pipe to hold the weights. Later, the apparatus can be used with one or two weight clamps. Finally, when you are ready, try lifting the apparatus with a weight held on by one of the clamps. It is

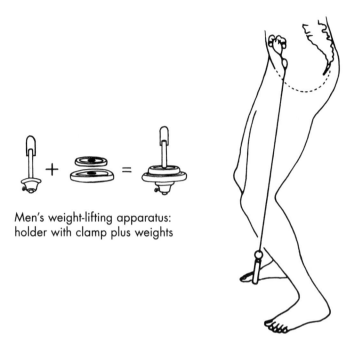

Men's weight-lifting apparatus:
holder with clamp plus weights

Fig. 3.5. Women can begin lifting by using the lifting apparatus alone.

better to lift lighter weights for longer periods than heavier weights for shorter periods. Never exceed one minute.

External Preparations

The room in which you practice should be quiet and well ventilated, but not cold. Keep a hard chair available for your meditation and as a place to rest the weight, unless you lift from the floor. The best time for these exercises is the morning after you shower and relieve your bladder and bowels. If you can, face the sun as you practice in the early morning hours, but never look directly into it at any time.

You are ready for Chi Weight Lifting practice when, after massaging the breasts and genitals, the vagina is moist with secretions. If not enough moisture is present, prepare the vagina with a natural lubricating cream. Women can feel reasonably safe with these practices—provided that the egg and string are kept sanitary—because the weight can be easily released if it proves too heavy to lift.

After learning how to use the egg, test yourself with the weight-holding apparatus before you add any weights to it. If it feels light to you, begin adding the weight clamps. Later, you may start adding standard weights. When you are ready, you can increase the weight until a maximum of 2½ pounds is reached. *Do not attempt to exceed this level on the first day.* Instead, try to sustain the weight for longer periods, but less than a minute, to release more energy.

Weight Lifting Goals

The Universal Healing Tao does not recommend anyone try to lift over 10 pounds without supervision. On the basis of this book 10 pounds should be considered the absolute maximum goal. Women may find that their lifting capabilities are slightly different than men's because they have no way to anchor the weight and are therefore more dependent upon internal power. It is certainly no shame for women to lift less than the 1 or 2 pounds recommended for beginners. If you choose to lift beyond 5 pounds, exercise more than the usual caution.

Warning: Lifting heaver weights without supervision is both foolish and contrary to the recommendations of this book. Further instruction in Bone Marrow Nei Kung is necessary for Chi Weight Lifting with heavier weights. Contact the Universal Healing Tao Center for information on advanced instruction.

PREPARATORY EXERCISES FOR CHI WEIGHT LIFTING

Chi Weight Lifting should be preceded and followed by both the Power Lock given in chapter 1 and the Sexual Energy Massage techniques, including the Cloth Massage, given in chapter 2.

Two additional practices should also precede Chi Weight Lifting: the Increasing Chi Pressure and Increasing Kidney Pressure exercises.

Increasing Chi Pressure

This exercise is done before the Power Lock exercise in order to ensure that the abdomen is full of chi.

1. Place the middle finger of each hand about 1½ inches below the navel at the lower tan tien (fig. 3.6).
2. Concentrate on the lower tan tien as you inhale chi into it, expanding the point with the resulting pressure. Your mental power will increase the energy flow to this area.

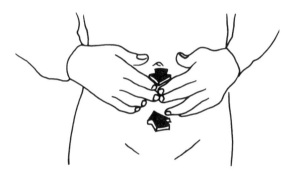

Fig. 3.6. Inhale and exhale up to 81 times to
the lower abdomen to increase chi pressure.
Use the fingers to press in.

 Increasing Kidney Pressure

1. Stand in a Horse stance with your feet slightly wider than shoulder width (see fig. 3.7 on page 92).
2. Rub your hands together until they are warm, and then apply their warmth to the kidneys by placing your energized palms on them from the back.
3. Bend your upper body forward slightly as you inhale, and pull up the left and right sides of the anus as you draw chi up to the kidneys.
4. Exhale, and deflate the kidneys.
5. Follow this sequence up to 36 times, and finish by warming the hands and again placing them on the kidneys.

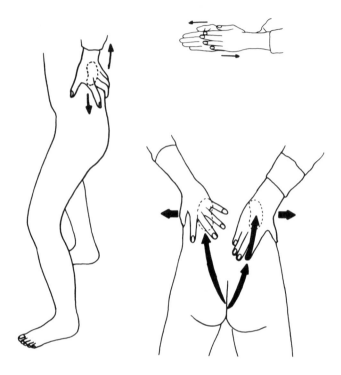

Fig. 3.7. Increasing Kidney Pressure

 Chi Weight Lifting

The Internal Egg Exercise described in chapter 2 can be used as a preparation for Chi Weight Lifting. During the actual lifting of weights, however, the egg is held deep inside the vaginal canal. Do not move it up and down, and do not release it.

Attaching the Weight

1. After the string has been passed through the egg and secured with a knot at the egg's large end, tie the weight to the string. The weight can also be placed inside a bag or container attached to the string. The weight holder prescribed for men can also be used, first without any weight, and then with the gradual addition of the holding clamp and then weight.

2. Either place a chair in front of you and rest the weight on it, or place the weight on the floor and squat down to facilitate the egg's insertion. (Remember to hold the weight with your fingers as you stand up.)

3. After you have massaged your breasts and vaginal areas in the prescribed manner, kneel down near where the weight is resting, and insert the egg into the vagina, large end first. (Use a lubricant if necessary.) Close the vagina, contracting the muscles around the egg to hold it (fig. 3.8).

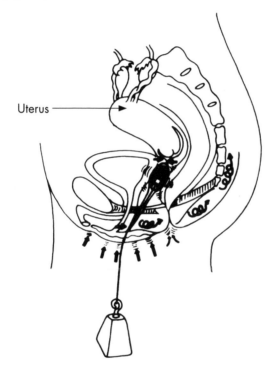

Uterus

Fig. 3.8. Contract the muscles around the egg to hold it.

☯ Testing and Lifting the Weight

1. Slowly stand up, holding the weight in your hand, and assume the Horse stance, with the feet parallel at about shoulder width, and the knees slightly bent. Use your index and middle fingers to test the weight and determine whether or not it is too heavy.

2. Inhale a sip of air and tightly close the external and internal vagina. At the same time, contract the uterus so that the vaginal canal is closed on both ends. As you inhale, squeeze the egg tightly, and pull it up until you feel you have gripped the egg firmly.

3. Slowly release the string from your fingers until you are holding the weight with the contracted muscles of the vagina. With the fingers of one hand nearby, feel the pull of the weight, and determine whether or not your vaginal muscles can sustain it. Do not remove your hand in case you did not grip the egg firmly enough. If the egg with the weight falls out you could be hurt.

4. Inhale as you contract the anus and perineum, then contract and hold first the lower and then the middle and upper vaginal muscles, so that the egg pushes deeply up into the vaginal canal. Start to pull from the cervix; feel the force of the cervix helping to pull up the weight. When you feel you are holding the egg and the weight securely, you are ready to rock the pelvis, thus swinging the weight (fig. 3.9).

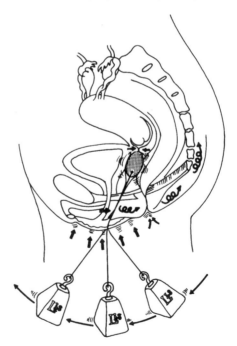

Fig. 3.9. Pulling from the cervix to hold the egg
securely for swinging the weight

☯ Swinging the Weight

Swinging the weight gives the practitioner control over the amount of pressure, which is why lighter weights are recommended. In the beginning swing the weights gently as you determine the amount of pressure that is comfortable for you.

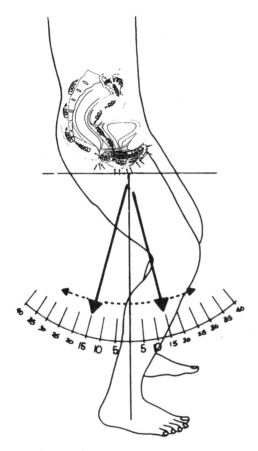

Fig. 3.10. Swing the weight at an angle between 15 and 30 degrees.

1. Swing the attached weight from 36 to 49 times (fig. 3.10). Pull up against the weight internally with each forward swing. Synchronize your breathing with each swing. Inhale as the weight swings forward, and exhale as it swings backward. Each completed swing back and forth should approximate 1 second. This will generate tremendous energy.

2. When you feel the energy build up, inhale slowly and deeply down to the ovaries, gathering your sexual energy, and carry it through the uterus and down to the clitoris. Hold it there.

3. Draw all the energy you have gathered up the spine and into the head, as you continue to hold the egg deeply inside of you. Still holding the same breath, continue gathering and pulling the sexual energy up into the head, where the brain can now be bathed in this wondrous nourishment.

4. Hold this energy in your brain, initially for 30 to 45 seconds, and gradually increasing the time as you feel ready.

5. Finally, put your tongue up to your palate, exhale, bring the energy down, and collect it at the navel.

6. To finish the practice, kneel as you place the weight on the chair or the floor again. Let the egg go, utilizing the contractile strength of the vaginal muscles to expel it. Disconnect the weight-holding apparatus.

7. After a week, try to swing the weight for 60 counts. More pressure results from the counterforce exerted by the Chi Muscle when heavier weights are swung, but rather than progressing rapidly to heavier weights, it is wiser to increase the pressure with lighter weights by adding more power to each swing. The lighter weights should be used to their maximum potential, thereby strengthening the Chi Muscle and producing more hormones.

☯ Finish with the Power Lock and Massage Techniques

1. Practice the Power Lock for at least 2 or 3 rounds after releasing the weight.

2. Then apply the Cloth Massage and the Sexual Energy Massage techniques.

3. Rest, and practice the Microcosmic Orbit meditation to circulate the tremendous energy you have generated, finally collecting it in the navel.

Lifting Weights from the Microcosmic Orbit

After you have practiced for 2 to 4 weeks, and feel comfortable with Chi Weight Lifting, begin to lift the weight from the stations of the Microcosmic Orbit. As you bring the chi up into the sacrum and higher centers, use this energy to pull the weight from each station. Take your time, and don't rush. Each point may require 1 or 2 weeks before you feel the flow of the Microcosmic Orbit working as part of the counterforce.

1. Sacrum: When you lift the weights suspended from the egg held by the contracted vaginal muscles, pull up the front, back, right, and left of the anus to bring the energy up to the sacrum (fig. 3.11). Hold it there. Breathe normally, and gently swing the weights. Feel a line of energy from the sexual center up to the sacrum.

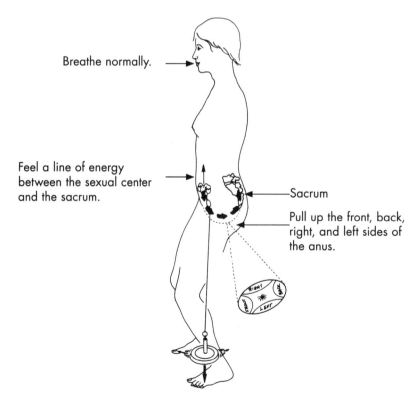

Fig. 3.11. Bring the energy up to the sacrum.

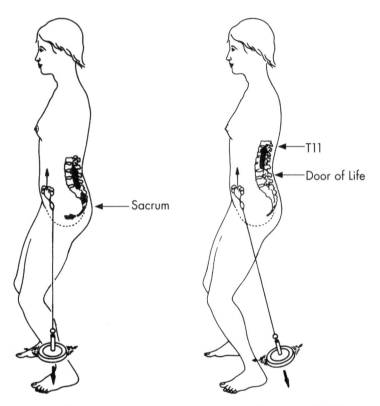

Fig. 3.12. From the sacrum bring the chi to the Door of Life (Ming Men).

Fig. 3.13. From the Door of Life bring the energy up to T11.

2. Door of Life: Once you feel the chi in the sacrum, bring it to the Door of Life on the spine, opposite the navel (fig. 3.12). Hold the chi there, and continue to swing the weights. Every time you swing, pull up more.

3. T11 point: From the Door of Life, bring the energy up to T11 on the spine, opposite the solar plexus (fig. 3.13). Feel the line of energy as it moves up to T11.

4. C7 point: Pull the energy from the sexual center, passing it through the sacrum, Door of Life, T11, and up to C7 at the base of the neck (fig. 3.14). Feel the line of energy from the sexual center up to C7.

5. Base of the skull: Next draw the chi through the sacrum, Door of Life, T11, and C7, and up to the base of the skull (fig. 3.15). Feel the line of chi flow from the sexual center up to the base of the skull.

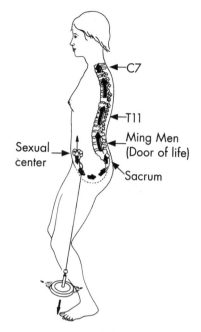

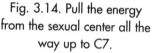

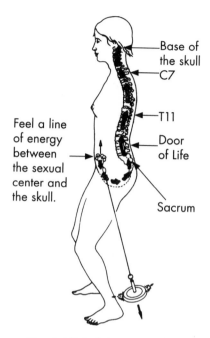

Fig. 3.14. Pull the energy from the sexual center all the way up to C7.

Fig. 3.15. Pull the energy from the sexual center all the way up to the base of the skull.

6. Crown point and the pineal gland: Draw the chi up to the Crown point where the pineal gland is (see fig. 3.16 on page 100). Remember that the sexual glands are closely related to the pineal and pituitary glands. You may feel this connection as these glands are stimulated.

7. The "third eye": Bring the chi to the third eye, or mid-eyebrow point, also called the "Crystal Room," where the pituitary gland is located (see fig. 3.17 on page 100).

8. With the tongue on the palate, bring the chi down to the throat center, the heart center, the solar plexus, and finally down to the navel (see fig. 3.18 on page 100). The overflow will spill back down to the sexual center.

9. At this point you have successfully brought the energy from the sexual center up through the spine, over the top of the head, down the front to the navel, and back again to the sexual center, circulating it through the Microcosmic Orbit. This process refines and enhances chi as it moves through the energy centers.

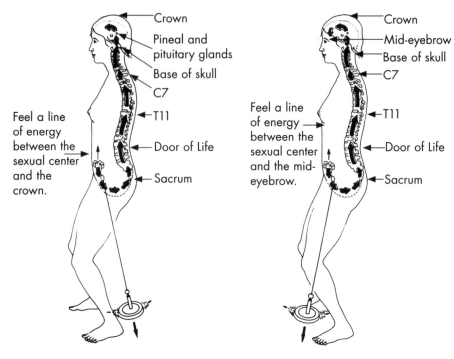

Crown
Pineal and pituitary glands
Base of skull
C7
T11
Door of Life
Sacrum

Feel a line of energy between the sexual center and the crown.

Fig. 3.16. Pull the energy from the sexual center all the way to the crown.

Crown
Mid-eyebrow
Base of skull
C7
T11
Door of Life
Sacrum

Feel a line of energy between the sexual center and the mid-eyebrow.

Fig. 3.17. Pull the energy from the sexual center all the way to the third eye.

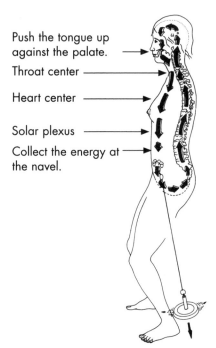

Push the tongue up against the palate.
Throat center
Heart center
Solar plexus
Collect the energy at the navel.

Fig. 3.18. Circulate the chi all the way around the Microcosmic Orbit and collect the energy at the navel.

10. Once the Microcosmic Orbit is open to the flowing sexual energy, all you need do is pull the energy up to the head, and then down to the navel through the tongue. Concentrate on drawing the energy up, circulating it in the Microcosmic Orbit, and storing it in the navel. The chi will flow very quickly through all the centers. You will no longer need to bring it up through the points of the spine one by one.

Advanced Chi Weight Lifting Using the Internal Organs

In this practice, once you have secured the egg in the vaginal canal, you pull with the higher organs and glands, which in turn pull on the lower organs and glands. They, in their turn, pull on the egg and weight.

Kidneys Help Pull the Weight

In the beginning stages of Chi Weight Lifting, it is the power of the kidneys that provides real internal counterforce (fig. 3.19). Once you can feel that power, it becomes easier to tap the force of the other organs to help lift

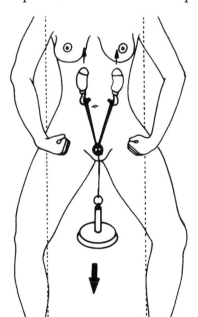

Fig. 3.19. In the beginning stages of Chi Weight Lifting it is the kidneys that provide the internal counterforce.

heavier weights. As you begin to increase the weight, start to use the strength of the other organs and glands to increase the upward counterforce. The main secret of internal power is to press the tongue against the roof of the mouth as you direct the force of the organ's energy toward it.

1. Always begin by pulling the energy up to the head several times to make sure of its flow within the Microcosmic Orbit.
2. Inhale with small sips, pull up the left side of the anus, and spiral the energy to the left kidney. Inhale again, pull up the right side of the anus, and spiral the energy into the right kidney (fig. 3.20). Hold the energy there, and feel the chi in the kidneys pull up toward the tongue, resisting the weight. Some people report that they can immediately feel the kidneys as they help lift the weight.
3. Exhale, maintaining the pulling action of the perineum and kidneys, and then breathe normally.

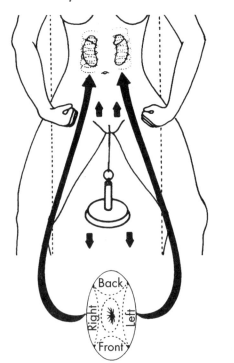

Fig. 3.20. When you feel the weight, inhale and pull up the right and left side of the anus. Wrap the energy around the kidneys.

🌀 Spleen and Liver Pull the Weight

Always keep the chest relaxed during these procedures. You can practice lifting from the spleen and liver as separate exercises or together as one exercise.

1. Spleen: Start again on the left side by pulling up the left side of the anus and perineum. Become aware of the spleen situated beneath the left side of the rib cage (fig. 3.21). (The spleen is located toward the back, slightly above the left kidney and adrenal gland.) Contract the left anus as you inhale a small sip of air. Pull the chi up to the spleen and left kidney with one more sip. Wrap the chi around and into the spleen. Keep the tongue pressed to the roof of your mouth. As you draw the chi in the spleen up toward the tongue, feel it help lift the weight.

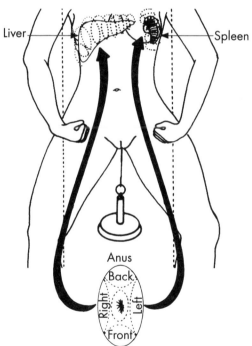

Fig. 3.21. Inhale and pull up the right side of the anus, directing the energy to the liver. Inhale and pull up the left side of the anus, directing the energy to the spleen. Wrap the energy around these organs.

2. Liver: Practice the same procedure on the liver, which lies under the right side of the rib cage. Pull up the right side of the anus and perineum. As you inhale, draw the chi up to the right kidney. Then become aware of your liver, and pull the chi up to it twice. Pack and wrap the liver with chi. Pull the energy toward the back, near the right kidney and adrenal gland. Push the tongue against the roof of your mouth. As you draw the chi in the liver up toward the tongue, feel it help lift the weight.

3. Combine the procedures of the spleen from the left side and the liver from the right side in order to help lift the weight. Pull their combined energies up toward the tongue.

❷ Lifting with the Lungs

Lifting a weight with the lungs is an advanced procedure and is more difficult than lifting with other organs and glands. Before you try to apply Chi Weight Lifting using the lungs, practice pulling energy up to each of the lower organs in succession, then drawing the organ energy up toward the tongue. Pull up the chi of the lower organs until you actually feel each lung contracting. Only lift with the lungs when you feel the energy reach them from the lower organs. Don't use force in this exercise. Use your chi to lift the weight in conjunction with light muscular contraction and strong mental power.

Each step should first be practiced separately. Later, all of the steps can be combined into one practice. The procedure is as follows.

1. First inhale and expand the upper left stomach near the left rib cage. Inhale again, and pull the stomach in toward the spine, up to the left rib cage, and then to the left lung. Push your left shoulder and side slightly toward the front.

2. Inhale a sip of air, pull up the left anus toward the left lung as you pull up the sexual organs. Pull up the left kidney, and then pull up the spleen. Feel the left kidney and the spleen assisting the left lung. Contract the muscles around the left lung, and draw the chi up to and around that lung through the lower organs (fig. 3.22).

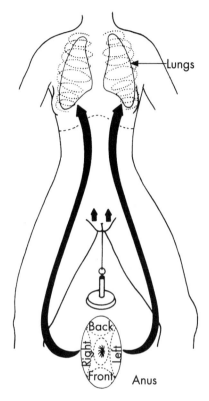

Fig. 3.22. Inhale and pull up both sides of the anus, directing the energy through the lower organs to the lungs. Wrap the energy around the lungs.

3. Pull the chi up from the left side of the anus to the bladder, left kidney, adrenal gland, and spleen until you feel the lung contracting. Feel all of these organs in a line between the lung and the sexual organs. Use the organs to pull up toward the tongue. Push your tongue hard against the roof of your mouth as you draw the chi up through the organs to the left lung.

4. Use the same procedure with the right side until a line can be felt passing through the associated organs, such as the right kidney and liver, to your right lung. When you feel the fascial connection to the sexual organs, use all of the lower organs to help lift the weight. Once you can exert this power from the lungs, you may eliminate the procedure of expanding the stomach area.

❂ *Lifting with the Heart (Cautiously!)*

As you progress to the heart, be sure that you are in control of the other organs first. The heart and lungs can easily become congested with energy, which can cause chest pain and difficult breathing. If you have this problem, tap the area around the heart and practice the healing sound of the heart. (The Six Healing Sounds are described in chapter 5 of this book and in *The Six Healing Sounds,* Destiny Books, 2009.)

Before lifting the weight, practice drawing up the chi and wrapping it into and around the heart. Proceed as follows with caution:

1. Create a ball of energy in the center of the abdomen, above the navel (fig. 3.23a).
2. Inhale a sip of air, pull up the front part of the anus, and expand the chi ball upward toward the rib cage (fig 3.23b).
3. Inhale another sip, draw the chi ball inward, and then pull it up under the sternum. Expand it under the sternum toward the back and to the left side.
4. Push your tongue up against the roof of your mouth, push the left shoulder toward the front, and feel your heart (fig. 3.23c).

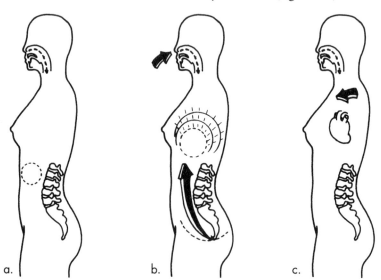

Fig. 3.23. Expanding a chi ball beneath the sternum

5. Slowly exhale, and regulate your breath.

6. When you are well practiced, eliminate the step of expanding the abdominal area. Simply inhale in sips, and pull up the front part of the anus as you pull up the sexual organs. Pull up the abdomen to the rib cage, and pull the chi to the heart, using the power of the heart. Wrap the chi into and around the heart.

7. Pull up the sexual organs, bladder, kidneys, liver, and spleen toward the tongue. Contract the muscles around the heart and lungs, and successively pull the chi up through each of the lower organs. Start lifting with the lower organs, and draw the chi upward through each of them to reach the heart.

8. When you are ready to practice Chi Weight Lifting from the heart, simply pull up the front part of the anus, the sexual organs, bladder, kidneys, liver, and spleen to the heart (fig. 3.24). Employ the power of the heart and lungs to help the other organs and glands lift the weight.

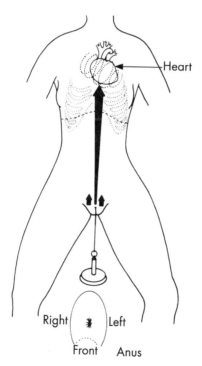

Fig. 3.24. Pull up the front part of the anus and direct the energy
to the heart. Wrap the energy around the heart.

◎ The Thymus Gland Adds Power to the Heart and Lungs

Contracting the muscles around the thymus, heart, and lungs will greatly increase their combined force.

1. First sink the sternum to the back and push the lungs toward the thymus under the sternum as you exhale.
2. Then connect the chi of the heart to the thymus, which is in close proximity to the heart. This will enable them to work together to draw chi up through the lower organs, pull up the genitals, and lift the weight (fig. 3.25).

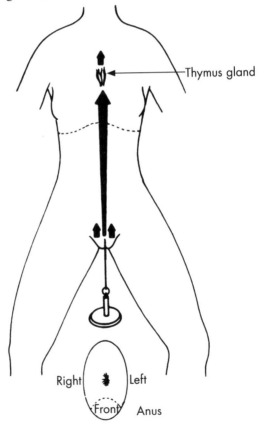

Fig. 3.25. Pull up the weight by contracting the thymus.

⊙ Pulling from the Pituitary and Pineal Glands

The tongue and eyes act as major tools in exerting control over the pituitary and pineal glands.

1. Practice this by first pressing the tongue to the palate and turning the eyes upward.
2. Then contract the eye muscles toward the middle of the brain and the pituitary gland.
3. Contract the cranium from all sides: Squeeze in from the crown, the base of the lower jaw near the throat, and the front, back, left, and right sides of the skull, gently compressing the center of the brain. Concentrating on the center point behind the mid-eyebrow, prepare to draw the energy up to the pituitary gland. You are using the muscles of the skull to increase the pressure on this area.
4. Contract the middle part of the anus, and pull the chi all the way up into the brain.
5. Contract the lungs, heart, and thymus gland, and push their energy up toward the center of the brain. The pituitary gland pulls energy from the thymus gland, heart, lungs, spleen, liver, adrenal glands, kidneys, bladder, and sexual organs. All of these parts will then work together to pull up the weight (see fig. 3.26 on page 110).
6. Repeat the practice, now focusing on the pineal gland at the crown of the head.

⊙ Circulate Energy through the Microcosmic Orbit

Since all the steps of this exercise are extremely powerful, use caution. After you have finished all of the steps mentioned above, circulate the energy in the Microcosmic Orbit several times, collecting it in the navel. This is a very important safety measure. Finally, remove the weight.

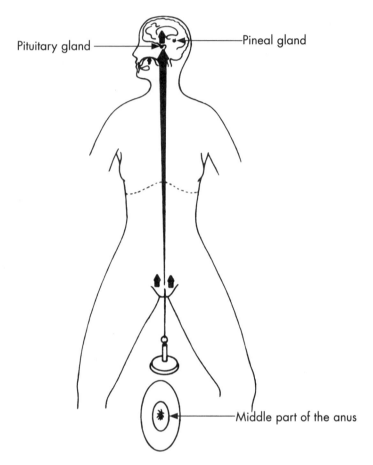

Pituitary gland

Pineal gland

Middle part of the anus

Fig. 3.26. Contract the middle part of the anus and pull up all the way to the brain. Lift the weight by contracting the pituitary gland.

❂ After Chi Weight Lifting

After you have released the weights, practice the Power Lock 2 or 3 times up to the crown, and massage the sexual organs again. First massage the genitals, sacrum, and perineum with the cloth, then practice the Sexual Energy Massage techniques. As stated earlier, the Universal Tao is not responsible for your use or misuse of this practice. The massage techniques are your best protection. Do not neglect them at any time.

PRECAUTIONS AND
SUGGESTIONS FOR PRACTICE

The best precaution is common sense. Read this section carefully to fully understand this practice!

1. Be sure that the Microcosmic Orbit is clear of any blockages.
2. Be well versed in all of the prerequisites before attempting this practice. Without the Six Healing Sounds, the organs may overheat. Without the Microcosmic Orbit meditation, there is no point in doing any practice taught in this system. Trouble would be the only result. Refer to chapter 5 for instructions in the Microcosmic Orbit and the Six Healing Sounds. Without a degree of mastery of Iron Shirt Chi Kung, which roots the body and draws energy from the earth, a student may not be grounded enough to safely accumulate external energies. Refer to *Iron Shirt Chi Kung* (Destiny Books, 2006) for the complete Iron Shirt practice.
3. If you have not mastered the Orgasmic Draw, do so before you practice Chi Weight Lifting. Refer to chapter 6 of *Healing Love Through the Tao* (Destiny Books, 2005) for detailed instruction in performing the Orgasmic Draw. Less chi will be available for the internal organs to pull the weight if too much sexual energy is expended. The remedy is not celibacy, but rather the practice of the Orgasmic Draw.
4. The ancient Taoist masters advised that one abstain from sex for the first one hundred days of this practice. For the best results in the modern world, abstain at least until you have comfortably mastered the lightest weights. Do not try to speed up your progress for this purpose. This is recommended because you must fully retain your sexual energy before you can safely practice Chi Weight Lifting.

   It is safe to practice Chi Weight Lifting after sex. You should still be prepared to reduce the weight, however, if the act of sex drains you in any way.

5. You should *never* practice Chi Weight Lifting during a menstrual period, vaginal infection, or at any stage of pregnancy. When these times have passed, practice may be resumed. Wait at least two or three days until after menstruation has finished.

6. Take extra care not to allow the accumulation of too much sexual energy in the head. Headaches, numbness, or discomfort can be alleviated by pressing the tongue to the roof of the mouth and drawing the pressure out of the head, down through the tongue, and into the navel. Spiral the energy, following the same procedures used at the end of the Microcosmic Orbit meditation.

7. Remember that the Ovarian Compression exercise is the best way to replenish the sexual energy you are extracting from the ovaries. Use this after the Chi Weight Lifting practice.

   Sexual energy transforms into life-force energy, which transforms into spiritual energy. The ability to stop the actual production of eggs means there is one less transformation for energy to go through, since life-force energy becomes directly available. This should not be taken to mean that such a practice is being advocated, but to inform you of its ramifications. The ancient masters saw this as a shortcut to the cultivation of spiritual energy, leaving one with fewer steps to cover on the spiritual path.

8. If you feel pain in your internal organs after training, practice the Microcosmic Orbit meditation and the Six Healing Sounds until the pain is gone. The pain may be a sign of overheating, which means that Chi Weight Lifting should be discontinued until the pain subsides. This may also be an indication that your internal organs are not in a healthy condition. If so, practice the less advanced techniques instead of Chi Weight Lifting until you can comfortably lift weights.

9. If you scratch the skin of the sexual area, clean the area, and allow it to heal before you do this practice. You may apply medications that you have used before, providing that the sexual organs are kept dry. (Hydrogen peroxide is useful for keeping a wound clean and dry.) See a physician or gynecologist for wounds within the vaginal

wall that require medication. Do not use any medications internally without a doctor's advice.

10. Although it is better to lift less weight for longer periods of time than to lift heavier weights for shorter periods, avoid lifting any weight for more than sixty seconds.

11. Do not try to outdo yourself or anyone else because you then stand a good chance of getting hurt. If you feel any strain at all, remove the weight immediately.

12. If you haven't practiced for more than a week, do not return to the same weight you were able to lift before the layoff. Build up again slowly to avoid injuring yourself.

13. When energy is low, and you still choose to practice, spend more time massaging the breasts and genitals and less time hanging the weight.

14. When some people detoxify, diarrhea, nausea, or pain in some of the organs may result as they are cleansed by the process. These are all temporary, however, Chi Weight Lifting (along with the Hitting practice) can also initiate some long-term effects that are ultimately good:

    • During the first hundred days of practice, a reduced sex drive may result from the transfer of sexual energy up to the higher centers to heal the organs and glands. Once the body has had a chance to repair itself, the sexual energy will increase greatly, thereby restoring the sex drive.

    • A need to drink more water may result from changes in metabolism.

    • Practice may cause either an increase or loss of appetite, accompanied by exhaustion. This may be part of the rebalancing process that the body goes through as energy is being assimilated. Some overweight people begin to lose weight; some underweight people find that they are eating more.

    • When you practice Chi Weight Lifting you may feel heat, muscle spasms, shakiness, coldness, breezes, or simply an overall "funny" feeling. The body may not yet be adjusted to the increase in chi,

or the energy may be fighting diseases in the body, thereby causing such symptoms. Use your own judgment as to whether you
should continue the process, but if serious physical problems
persist, consult your doctor.

- As certain levels of practice are attained, some people dream
profusely. This may be because they are practicing Chi Weight
Lifting and Hitting in excess, or they may be hitting too hard.
This causes the organs to overheat. Also, if the physical body is
too hard and tight, emotions may be locked in the muscles and
organs. The Hitting process may release them. Pain felt in the
tendons and muscles can cause a great deal of dreaming. The
increase in chi, and its fight against diseases of the body, can
cause great internal changes, which may also be the source of
excessive dreaming.

15. Be especially careful if you suffer from high blood pressure.
Concentrate on opening your Microcosmic Orbit. Once it is
open and flowing, blood pressure can be reduced and eventually
controlled.

16. Do not practice Chi Weight Lifting on a full stomach. Wait at least
one hour after a meal before practicing. Also, to keep from losing
chi when you have finished exercising, do not eat for one-half hour
to an hour.

17. Do not shower right away after practice, especially if you sweat.
Allow your body to cool down for a while. You are still absorbing
chi at this point; therefore, it is better to avoid washing away external
energy.

18. Urinate or have a bowel movement before practice. If this is not
possible, try to wait one or two hours after practice before fulfill-
ing these functions in order to prevent any loss of accumulated
chi. This will give the body time to absorb the chi into the bones,
organs, and glands. Collect the energy in the navel.

19. In hot weather, do not drink too much cold water because the body
must expend a great deal of internal energy to warm it. This may
result in too much cold energy in the heart, which can be harmful.

20. Many people have reported a loss of desire for alcohol, drugs, tobacco, coffee, and tea as a result of the detoxification initiated by Chi Weight Lifting. It is best to avoid these toxic substances in any case, but keep in mind that they will satisfy you less if you detoxify faster than these substances are taken in. The stimulation they offer may not occur if they are forced out of the body before they can affect you.

21. Do not stand on a cold floor during practice. If there is no rug, stand on a towel. A cold floor will draw away your energy.

22. In the early stages, avoid practicing at night, because you may not be able to sleep. When you become proficient, you should be able to practice at any time.

23. Remember that the purpose of your training is to raise your energy levels and to rid your body of toxins. It is *not* to promote violence or foolishness. Do not walk into your local bar and make claims to being "the sexual weight-lifting champion of the Universal Healing Tao." You may find that this particular subject is not well received in certain social atmospheres.

24. Be aware that practices that draw sexual energy into the body can spread any existing venereal infection. Be sure that you are free of such problems before attempting the Sexual Energy Massage or Chi Weight Lifting.

Warning: Be aware of your body's reactions to Chi Weight Lifting. Although this system is known for its many safeguards for avoiding side effects, it is difficult to account for the internal differences in people. *Any* problems that do not appear to be covered in this book must be directed to the Universal Healing Tao. In such cases, Chi Weight Lifting should be discontinued until you are fully aware of your status.

4

Cleansing, Detox, and Nutrition

To assist in balancing your energy and maintaining your health you need to open up and clean out what are known as the front and back doors of the body. In addition, proper nutrition supports health and strength in every way and following certain nutritional guidelines can be particularly effective in cancer prevention.

THE BACK DOOR
The Colon

The key to the health of the back door, and in many ways the health of the whole body, is how well you eliminate the toxins and built-up debris you have ingested. For the colon—which includes the anus, rectum, and the whole lower abdomen—Taoists highly recommend regular cleansing practices to clear out any buildup of toxins. The most important of these practices are colonics and dry skin brushing; also recommended are rectum cleansing, a natural-sponge face wash, and solar bathing. These cleansing practices are described in more detail below.

In general, breathing deeply and mindfully—by expanding the lower abdominals to draw air in and thus expand the lungs, and then flattening the abdominals to push the used air out of the body—helps to activate and repair all of the body's natural eliminative processes. In this way, any type of aerobic exercise will help elimination by activating the lungs, which then activate their paired organ, the colon. Conversely, when you clean out the back door you will also improve your breathing.

If you have never cleaned out your colon or rectum, and have been building up toxins for twenty or thirty or forty years, you can just imagine what is in there. You need to cleanse this area of the body just as you do the other end of the body (the mouth and the teeth). As you cleanse the colon you will start to eliminate a lot of excess body fat and acids.

Colonics

Colonics are a method of flushing the colon with water to clear out impacted food waste and debris. There are two main types of colonics— an open-ended type and a closed-end type. The open-ended colonic involves the insertion into the rectum of a thin-tipped hose, which is connected to a container filled with lukewarm water. Other ingredients, known as implants, might be added to the water, including chlorophyll, coffee, garlic, Epsom salts, or a combination of these. A closed-end colonic device is operated by a colon therapist. Its metal insert sends water into the colon and pulls the evacuated debris out.

The process of a colonic is similar to a mouthwash, except that it happens in the colon. You wash the internal skin of the colon and thereby release any blockages. But whereas the closed-end type uses a machine to push water in and flush it back out, the open-ended type relies on gravity and the actual rectal muscles to eliminate the water solution and its accompanying debris. In this book we will be describing methods and practices for open-ended colonics that you can do at home; if you prefer, however, you can have them performed at a professional facility instead (see fig. 4.1 on page 118).

A colonic series consists of one colonic every other day for a week to two weeks. You should do a series every six months to cleanse out your whole body. The only caution is that colonics will draw out from the digestive wall a lot of the natural bacteria that you need to digest food;

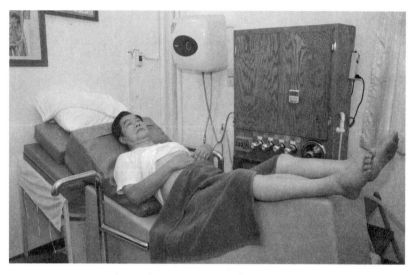

Fig. 4.1. Colonic cleansing at a professional colonic facility

you will need to include acidophilus supplements so you can culture the bacteria again within the colon.

With an open-ended colonic you will fill up a bucket of water, put it over the toilet to give it gravity, and sit on a special board as you hook tubing up over the toilet.* As you slowly release water from the tip of the bucket tubing into the rectum, you can massage your abdomen and also do light aerobic exercises to help your body eliminate (figs. 4.2 and 4.3).

One of the problems with the colon is that human beings stand upright—unlike other animals, who are on all fours. Because of our upright stance, our bodies have to move waste up the body in the ascending colon, against gravity. This means that someone with deficient chi may become constipated, further exacerbating any unhealthy condition. Once you are cleaning your colon regularly you will start to realize that how you defecate is important. Odors, gas, and even the way you sit become important details of your daily life. If you have a very cleansing diet that includes a lot of chlorophyll, for instance, there will be no smell at all to defecation, or any gas either. Much of the gas and the smells we

---

*See the resource section at the end of the book for sources of colonic boards, tubing, and other necessary colonic supplies.

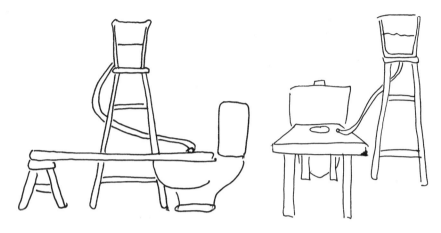

Fig. 4.2. Set-up for an open-ended colonic
that can be self-administered

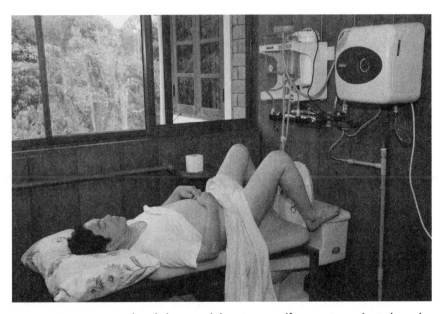

Fig. 4.3. Massaging the abdomen while using a self-operating colonic board

associate with our bowels actually come from improper foods that do not agree with the body. It is the horrible combinations of what we put into our bodies—the animal products, the acidic products, the sugars, and starches—that create a chemical reaction as they start to break down; this leads to explosions of gas.

The best position for defecating is a squatting posture. In much of Asia, they do not have toilet seats because they squat on their haunches instead. This is a much more hygienic method because you do not physically sit on anything, so there is no risk of germ transmission. Many traditional Asian cultures also use water to wash the anus instead of toilet paper, which has a tendency to get matted up in the buttocks and prevent proper drying.

Colonic Cleansing

1. Set colonic board hood on toilet and board on stool or use a professional colonic specialist.
2. Hook up tubing to bucket; then fill it with warm water and rinse. Check water release.
3. Insert rectal tip into tube in board hood. Place pad on board and lie on your back on the board with your buttocks on the hood.
4. Apply rectal gel and insert rectal tip into anus.
5. Relax. Release tube clamp. Allow water to flow freely.
6. Massage the left side of your lower abdomen—the descending colon—in an upward direction (against its normal direction of flow) toward the bottom of the rib cage. Work through any tender spots. Continue across the transverse colon just below the rib cage, and then down the right side, which is the ascending colon.
7. When it becomes necessary to evacuate, relieve the bowels by expelling water. Feces will normally bypass the tip without pushing it out.
8. Repeat steps 5–7 a few times until the bucket is empty (about 45 minutes). Do not flush the toilet during the entire colonic. Instead, look at what comes out (it will be black/green feces).
9. To finish, clamp the tube, remove the tip, and slip out from the board. Wash the board; then sit on the toilet to defecate.
10. Clean yourself; then collect energy at your navel point as follows. Starting at the navel, spiral the energy outward in a clockwise direction, making 36 revolutions. Once you have completed the clockwise revolutions, spiral inward in a counterclockwise direction 24 times, ending and collecting the energy at the navel.

Do 2 colonics per day for 7 days, or 1 colonic every other day for 2 weeks.

Implants

Implants are additives that are placed in the water during a colonic. They can be used to nourish the body and aid cleansing. They can be combined or used individually.

- Chlorophyll liquid concentrate (½ cup of liquid squeezed from green grass)
- Coffee (2 tablespoons ground coffee simmered in 1 quart of water for 15 minutes, strained and added to bucket)
- Garlic (3 cloves blended and strained into bucket)
- Lemon juice (¼ cup strained into bucket)
- Saline (1 tablespoon of sun-dried sea salt dissolved into bucket)
- Epsom salts (1 tablespoon dissolved into bucket)
- Glycothymoline (8 ounces per 5 gallons of water)
- Acidophilus (1 quarter of bottle into bucket)

After your colonic series ends, eat only whole fruits and vegetables for 2 days. They can be steamed or cooked into soup. Also take acidophilus twice a day for 2 weeks.

Dry Skin Brushing

In Chinese medicine, the skin is often called a "third lung" because of its connection to the lungs and large intestine. For this reason, a colon cleanse also includes opening and cleaning out the pores of the skin with dry skin brushing and solar bathing. Skin brushing should be done on a regular basis for maintenance, youthfulness, and longevity, and should be included in the periodic colon cleanse (see fig. 4.4 on page 122).

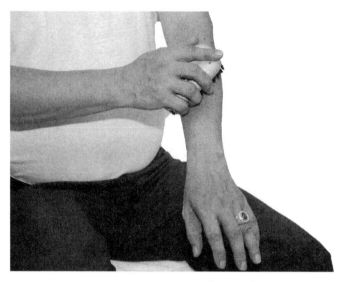

Fig. 4.4. Dry Skin Brushing

Use a bristle brush or loofah brush before your morning bath and before bed at night. Gently brush with strokes from outer points of the body to the center. The skin should glow with a pink color; it should not turn red. The total process takes about 3 minutes.

1. Do the Inner Smile meditation (see chapter 5 for directions on how to do the Inner Smile meditation).
2. Beginning at the sole of the right foot, brush from sole of foot up the entire leg to the groin. Use short, quick strokes or long, sweeping strokes toward the heart. Use as many strokes as are needed to brush the front, back, and sides of the leg.
3. Repeat step 2 on the left leg.
4. Brush buttocks, hips, lower back, and abdomen with circular motions.
5. Brush the left arm from the hand up to the shoulder, then circle the left breast. Make sure to brush the top, bottom, and sides of the arm.
6. Repeat step 5 on the right arm and breast.
7. Brush across the upper back, then down the front, back, and sides of the torso. Cover entire skin surface once.
8. Use a softer brush on the face. Begin in the center of the face and stroke outward. Brush down the sides of the face and neck.

9. To finish, jump into the shower and feel a light, tingling sensation over your body.

10. Clean and dry your body, then collect energy at the navel point as follows. Starting at the navel, spiral the energy outward in a clockwise direction, making 36 revolutions. Once you have completed the clockwise revolutions, spiral inward in a counterclockwise direction 24 times, ending and collecting the energy at the navel.

 ## Rectum Cleansing

After defecating on the toilet, it's a good time to clean the rectum. You will need the following supplies: a surgical glove or plastic finger cot, castor oil, Dr. Bronner's pure castile soap.

1. While sitting on the toilet after completing your bowel movement, cover your middle finger with a finger cot or surgical glove and insert it into your rectum. Clean out your rectum, massaging the upper roof of the rectum wall, which will effectively massage the uterus.

2. Remove your finger, keeping the finger cot on, and apply castor oil. Re-insert the finger into your rectum and clean again. It may take several rounds of cleaning to complete the process, as you are likely to experience a few more bowel movements while you do it.

3. Remove the glove and clean your hands with pure castile soap.

 ## Natural Sponge Face Wash

You can perform this facial wash any time your skin feels tight or dry. When done on a regular basis it can prevent dry skin and signs of aging. You will need a natural sea sponge and cool purified water for this practice.

1. Soak the sea sponge in purified water and gently apply it to your face (see fig. 4.5 on page 124). You can gently clean, rub, and massage your skin.

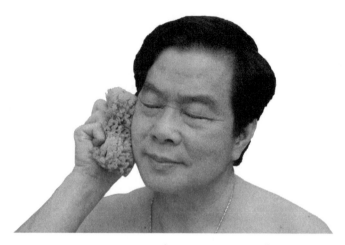

Fig. 4.5. Natural Sponge Face Wash

2. After completing the wash do not dry your face. Instead, allow it to dry naturally, so that your facial skin will absorb the purified water.

 Solar Bathing

If you are lucky enough to have a sunny area with some privacy, you will probably enjoy this practice (fig 4.6). The sun's energy is very healing and soothing to the genitals and can be absorbed by the ovaries through the genitals.

1. The best time of day to practice solar bathing is in the early morning (between 7 and 9 a.m.) and in the late afternoon (between 3 and 5 p.m.).
2. If you lie on your back, place your hands under your waist, palms down, thumbs touching, and place the soles of the feet together. This position completes the energy circulation through the hands and feet.
3. Before you begin, massage the mons area and along the outer lips. Open the labia to the sun and use your mind to draw the solar energy into your ovaries. Let this energy mix with your own energy as you circulate it in the Microcosmic Orbit (see chapter 5 for directions on the how to do the Microcosmic Orbit meditation).

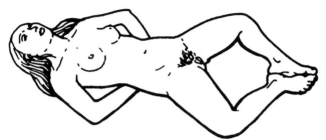

Palms down, thumbs touching, soles of the feet touching

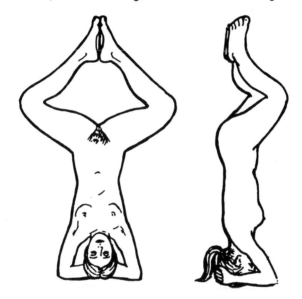

Fig. 4.6. Solar bathing—absorbing yang energy

4. Sun for no more than 5 minutes in the beginning, eventually working up to 10 minutes.

Cellular Cleansing

While you are doing a colonic cleanse, we suggest you do a cellular cleanse at the same time to improve your results. This cleanse consists of a 7- to 14-day fast, during which you ingest only vegetable broths and specific herbs and supplements. These supplements will activate your energy and help to loosen the debris in your system, so that it is more easily removed by the colonics.

This cellular cleanse came from natural health pioneer Victor Irons over ninety years ago; it recommends oral bentonite and psyllium for cleansing the colon, and taking supplements to strengthen and build up the cells. Together, the supplements—including chlorophyll, digestive enzymes, and essential fatty acids—draw toxins out of individual cells and into the intestinal system, where they can be effectively eliminated. Then psyllium and bentonite help to pull the debris off of the colon walls, which allows you to eliminate this caked up material from your body.

Bentonite is a form of clay that was once blown into the sky by volcanic action, then sifted down to earth, where it collected in layers or veins that can be mined. Its action is due to three things. First, its large and varied mineral content gives it a negative electrical charge, which attracts positively charged particles. In the human body, much of the toxic poisons are positively charged. Second, the minuteness of the particles of bentonite give it a very large surface area in proportion to its volume, thus enabling it to pick up many times its own weight in positively charged particles such as body acid debris. Third, to obtain maximum effectiveness in the human body, it should be in a liquid colloidal gel state. For information on where to buy colloidal bentonite and the other supplements recommended in this cleanse, see the resource section at the end of this book.

Clays have been used as natural medicines for thousands of years. Nutrition pioneer Weston A. Price found clay in common use among the Yucatan Indians of Mexico, for instance. When an Indian had a cut, bruise, abrasion, or irritation, he would immediately make a "mudpie" with a particular clay and apply it to the affected area to help it heal. The Yucatan people also took clay internally; when they did not feel "up to par" generally, they would immediately mix a special clay into a solution with water and drink it. This seemed to relieve whatever symptoms were present, and in a great many cases, these people seemed to live to a ripe old age.

Indigenous people from places as diverse as the Andes, Central Africa, and Australia have also been known to ingest clay. In many cases people regularly dipped their food into clay to prevent a "sick stomach."

The Cellular Cleanse (with Colonics)

This is a liquid fasting cell cleanse that uses bentonite, psyllium, and various supplements for a period of 7 to 14 days, with a colonic every other day for greatest results. You should eat nothing for the 7 to 14 days of the cleanse, but you may drink herbal teas or vegetable broths.

Note that you should always consult your physician about your ability to complete this cleanse. If you are able, we recommend that you do this cleanse 2 to 4 times a year.

You will need the following supplies for this cleanse: a pint jar, apple juice, apple cider vinegar, honey, bentonite, psyllium seed husks, and the supplements listed in the table below. Sources for purchasing these supplements are listed in the resource section. You will also need the colonic supplies listed in the resource section.

The cleanse consists of two drinks mixed separately. Drink them in succession 5 times per day.

First Drink

Place all of the ingredients in jar. Shake for 15 seconds. Drink quickly.

> 2 ounces apple juice, lemon juice, or lime juice for
>   flavor
> 8 ounces pure water
> 1 tablespoon colloidal bentonite
> 1 teaspoon psyllium

Second Drink

Place all ingredients in pint jar. Shake, and drink quickly.

> 10 ounces pure water
> 1 tablespoon apple cider vinegar or other vinegar
> 1 teaspoon honey or pure maple syrup

⚛ Supplements

Along with the two cleansing drinks, you will need to take the supplements listed in the table below 4 times a day on the days specified. You should separate the cleansing drinks and the supplements by 1½ hours. For example, if you take the cleansing drinks at 7:00 a.m., you should take the supplements at 8:30.

SUPPLEMENT SCHEDULE (4 TIMES PER DAY)

	Day 1	Day 2	Days 3, 7, 14
Chlorophyll gel tablets	12	18	24
Vitamin C tablets	200mg	200mg	800mg
Pancreatic enzyme tablets	6	6	6
Beet tablets	2	2	2
Dulse tablets	1	1	1
Enzymatic tablets	2	2	2
Niacin tablets	50mg	100mg	200mg
Wheat germ oil tablets	1	1	1

THE FRONT DOOR

The Urinary Tract and Genitals

For the urinary tract, which includes the vagina, ovaries, bladder, and kidneys, most of the cleansing practices focus on the kidneys. As the source of sexual energy, the kidneys are a vital energy center that needs to be kept in good health. To help to keep the kidneys clean and in prime condition, Taoists highly recommend herbal teas, vegetable cleanses, and Sexual Energy Massage on a regular basis. These will help to clear out any debris, blockages, and built-up toxins from the urinary tract. Vaginal douches can also be helpful.

Cleansing the Kidneys

The kidneys are extremely delicate, blood-filtering organs that congest easily. Dehydration, poor diet, weak digestion, stress, and an irregular lifestyle can all contribute to the formation of kidney stones. Most kidney grease/crystals/stones, however, are too small to be detected through modern diagnostic technology, including ultrasounds or X-rays. They are often called "silent" stones and do not seem to bother people much. When they grow larger, though, they can cause considerable distress and damage to the kidneys and the rest of the body.

To prevent kidney problems and kidney-related diseases, it is best to eliminate kidney stones before they can cause a crisis. You can easily detect the presence of sand or stones in the kidneys by pulling the skin under your eyes sideways toward the cheekbones. Any irregular bumps, protrusions, red or white pimples, or discoloration of the skin indicates the presence of kidney sand or kidney stones.

Herbal Kidney Cleanse

The following herbs, when taken daily for a period of 20 to 30 days, can help to dissolve and eliminate all types of kidney stones, including uric acid, oxalic acid, phosphate, and amino acid stones. If you have a history of kidney stones, you may need to repeat this cleanse a few times, at intervals of 6 weeks (see page 130 for directions).

Marjoram (1 ounce)
Cat's claw (1 ounce)
Comfrey root (1 ounce)
Fennel seed (2 ounces)
Chicory herb (2 ounces)
Uva ursi (2 ounces)
Hydrangea root (2 ounces)
Gravel root (2 ounces)
Marshmallow root (2 ounces)
Goldenrod herb (2 ounces)

✪ Directions

1. Thoroughly mix all the herbs together and put them in an airtight container. You may put them in the refrigerator.
2. Before bedtime, put 3 tablespoons of the herb mixture in 2 cups of water. Cover, and let it sit overnight.
3. The following morning, bring the concoction to a boil; then strain it. (If you forget to soak the herbs in the evening, boil the mixture in the morning and let it simmer for 5 to 10 minutes before straining.)
4. Drink a few sips at a time in 6 to 8 portions throughout the day. This tea does not need to be taken warm or hot, but do not refrigerate it. Also, do not add sugar or sweeteners. Wait at least 1 hour after eating before taking your next sips.
5. Repeat this procedure for 20 days.

If you experience discomfort or stiffness in the area of the lower back, this is because mineral crystals from kidney stones are passing through the ducts of the urinary system. Normally, the release is gradual and does not significantly change the color or texture of the urine, but any strong smell or darkening of the urine that occurs during the kidney cleanse indicates a major release of toxins from the kidneys.

Note: Support your kidneys during this cleanse by drinking extra amounts of water, a minimum of 6 to 8 glasses per day. However, if the urine is a dark yellow color, you will need to drink more than that amount.

Bone Marrow Soup
Kidney Cleanse

Make a bone marrow soup with the following ingredients, and drink it on a regular basis to maintain kidney performance and health.

Cracked organic beef bone (knuckles),
marrow exposed

Seaweed (hijiki or nori)
Garlic
Added vegetables: Carrots, onions, zucchini,
celery, burdock root, daikon radish

Kidney Tonics

The following preparations tone the kidneys and increase their ability to filter impurities from the blood.

Cranberry juice (unsweetened) with an equal
amount of purified water
1 to 2 lemons juiced in purified water

Vaginal Douching

A douche is a device used to introduce a stream of water into the vagina for medical or hygienic reasons. Douche usually refers to vaginal irrigation, the rinsing of the vagina, but it can also refer to the rinsing of any body cavity. The word *douche* comes from the French language, in which its principal meaning is "shower" (the French phrase for vaginal douching is *douche vaginale,* meaning "vaginal shower"). A douche bag is a piece of equipment for douching—a bag for holding the fluid used in douching. Today a vaginal bulb syringe is often used. To avoid transferring intestinal bacteria into the vagina, the same bag or syringe must not be used for a vaginal douche and an enema.

Vaginal douches may consist of water, water mixed with vinegar, garlic, acidophilus, or even antiseptic chemicals. Douching has been touted as having a number of supposed but unproven benefits. In addition to promising to clean the vagina of unwanted odors, it can also be used by women who wish to avoid smearing a sexual partner's penis with menstrual blood while having intercourse during menstruation.

Please do vaginal douching at your own discretion, as it can interfere with both the vagina's normal self-cleaning and with the natural bacterial culture of the vagina, which could lead to irritation, bacterial vaginosis, and pelvic inflammatory disease (PID). Frequent douching with water may result in an imbalance of the pH of the vagina, and thus may put women at risk for possible yeast infections.

OPTIMUM NUTRITION
FOR HEALTH

The three vital functions of food are to rebuild the living tissues, to supply energy, and to preserve a proper medium in which the biochemical processes of the body can take place. To ensure that all three take place, it is important to follow twelve rules of healthful eating.

1. Eat only when hungry and stop before you are full.
2. Maintain proper balance of acid and alkaline and yin and yang.
3. Chew your food well and mix thoroughly with saliva.
4. Refrain from eating when emotionally upset or physically exhausted.
5. Eat food at room temperature.
6. Eat fresh natural organic raw and cooked foods daily.
7. Fast or follow an eliminative diet when necessary.
8. Combine food properly.
9. Refrain from close eye work or intense brain work before, during, or after meals.
10. Eat your last meal at least three to four hours before bedtime.
11. Be cheerful and calm at mealtime.
12. Follow the law of moderation.

An elaboration of all twelve keys to good health, along with extensive nutritional guidance for health and longevity, can be found in our book, *Cosmic Nutrition* (Destiny Books, 2012). Here we focus on maintaining an alkaline-based diet, necessary to achieve the optimum results from the Chi Kung exercises for women's health.

Balancing Acid and Alkaline

In order to grasp the significance of acid and alkaline, we must first understand the meaning of pH, which is a measure of hydrogen ion concentration in blood, urine, and liquids, and is used as symbol to indicate acidity and alkalinity. A pH of 7 (.0000001 gram atom of hydrogen ion per liter) is considered neutral, the measure of pure water. The acid end of the pH scale is from 1 to 7, and 7 to 14 is the alkaline end. In the human body, a slightly alkaline blood and lymph is a requirement for health and long life.

Solvent type foods such as watery fruits, juices, and nonstarchy vegetables are alkaline. The heavier type foods are acid: all proteins, starches, fats, and sugars, that is, all nuts, seeds, cheeses, bread, potatoes, rice, oils, dried and sweet fruit (like dates, raisins, figs, bananas), and so on.

All ripe fruits are alkaline-reacting within the system. These alkalines neutralize the acid poisons, uric acid, and acidosis, which usually come from a high-protein meat diet. In addition, according to Chi Kung master Jeff Primack, in his book *Conquering Any Disease,* ellagic acid, which is considered to be a cancer inhibitor, is found in forty-six different fruits. Its richest source is raspberries.

Cancer Inhibitors

In *Conquering Any Disease,* Jeff Primack also specifically recommends certain other foods for their support of overall health and cancer prevention:

- Asparagus, which boasts the highest glutathione levels of any food, glutathione being unmatched in its ability to remove poisons from the body.
- *Agaricus blazei,* a mushroom with legendary immune system benefits.
- Black beans aid kidney functioning and sexual disorders.
- Kidney beans are also said to strengthen the kidneys; in addition they are rich in protein and very warming and nourishing.

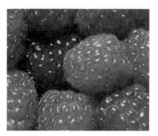

Raspberries

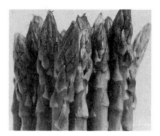

Asparagus

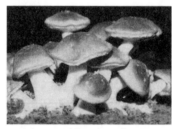

Agaricus blazei mushrooms

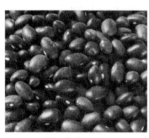

Black beans

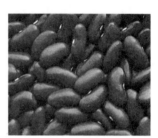

Kidney beans

Fig. 4.7. Health power foods

As explained by Lino Stanchion in his book *Power Eating Program,* for cancer prevention foods need to be chewed completely for maximum results and benefits. In addition to promoting a more alkaline condition in the body, chewing activates and balances all the glands, from the pituitary and thyroid to the pancreas, spleen, and ovaries.

Another route is that suggested by Primack in *Conquering Any Disease* and *Smoothie Formulas,* in which foods are taken in smoothie form, such as in the Alkalizer Smoothie recipe shown on page 135.

The Alkalizer Smoothie

Blend together:

1½ cup distilled water
3 stalks of organic celery
½ organic cucumber
½ lime with pith and seeds
1 Fuji apple sliced with skin and seeds
3 leaves of Swiss chard
1 node of cilantro

Special Recipes to Tone the Ovaries

Women who have any weakness in their sexual organs may wish to try the following simple and delicious recipes.

Strengthening Tonic for the Ovaries

To gradually increase energy flow in the ovaries, try the following mixture.

1 cup whiskey
1 cup honey
1 cup lemon juice

Directions

1. Combine the ingredients and stir well until the honey dissolves. Drink 1 to 2 tablespoons daily.
2. Store the mixture in a previously sterilized jar in a cool dry place. Shake the jar well before each use. This recipe will last several months. The more it ages, the better it becomes.

Caution: If you are experiencing a very heavy menstrual flow, refrain from taking the mixture for a few days, until the flow has normalized.

Chicken or Vegetarian Soup
with Dong Quai

An herb with numerous valuable properties, dong quai (*Angelica sinensis*) should be an integral component of a woman's health care regimen. Because it is loaded with good nutrition for the ovaries and hormones, women can benefit from this herb throughout their lifetimes. It is especially good as a blood tonic, being quite rich in iron, and it is excellent for alleviating a variety of menstrual problems. You can obtain dong quai in Chinese herb stores located in every Chinatown. Such stores often have mail order services. The herb may also be purchased in many natural food stores.

1. To make the soup, simply place 1 to 2 pieces of the herb (about 1 inch in size each) in chicken broth or soup, and season as desired. Simmer in a slow cooker for approximately 3 to 5 hours. Vegetarians can make dong quai soup in the same manner, using the slow cooker and a meatless broth.
2. Take dong quai only 1 to 2 times per month, and only after the menstrual cycle has ended, never during the cycle. After using dong quai on a regular basis for a 1- or 2-month period, you will notice a definite increase in your strength.

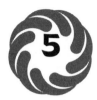

Summary of Chi Kung Practices for Women's Health and Sexual Vitality

The exercises and practices in this book are meant to enhance and heal the body's sexual energies through Chi Kung for the prevention of any type of gynecological cancer while rejuvenating your sexual vitality. In addition to the exercises summarized below, your health and vitality will be supported by the cosmic detox and nutritional practices detailed in chapter 4.

You should proceed with caution and patience when doing these Chi Kung practices, allowing the body to respond in a timely manner.

Chi Kung Daily Practices for Women:

1. Inner Smile
2. Microcosmic Orbit
3. Six Healing Sounds
4. Ovarian Breathing
5. Ovarian Compression
6. Bone Breathing

7. Bone Compression
8. Increasing Chi and Kidney Pressure
9. Power Lock
10. Sexual Energy Massage
11. Internal Egg Exercise
12. Chi Weight Lifting

These practices are described here in a condensed format so you can practice them using these pages as guidelines to help you master the formulas of Chi Kung for women's health and sexual vitality.

PREPARATION:
INNER SMILE AND MICROCOSMIC ORBIT

The energy from your mother that formed your body entered it through the umbilical cord, then moved from the navel down to the sacrum, then up the spine to the crown (Governing Channel), then down the front of the body (Functional Channel), back to the navel. As long as you are alive your energy moves within this Microcosmic Orbit. Once you become aware of this flowing energy, you can use it to heal any internal energy blockage in your body.

The Microcosmic Orbit meditation is initiated by the practice known as the Inner Smile, which draws positive energy to the internal organs and glands. For both, sit on the edge of a chair with your hands held together and eyes closed. Full descriptions of these practices can be found in *The Inner Smile* (Destiny Books, 2008) and *Healing Love through the Tao* (Destiny Books, 2005).

The Inner Smile

Front Line: The Functional Channel

1. Be aware of smiling cosmic energy in front of you and breathe it into your eyes.

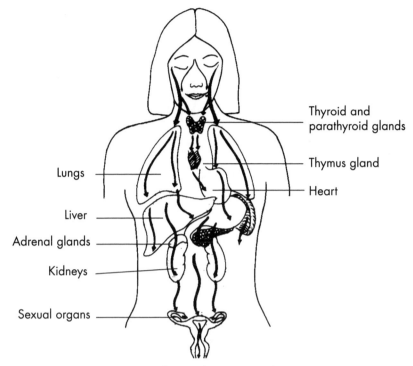

Thyroid and
parathyroid glands

Thymus gland

Lungs

Heart

Liver

Adrenal glands

Kidneys

Sexual organs

Fig. 5.1. Front line smile: major vital organs

2. Allow smiling energy to enter the point between your eyebrows. Let it flow into your nose and cheeks, and let it lift up the corners of your mouth, bringing your tongue to rest on your palate.
3. Smile down to your neck, throat, thyroid, parathyroid, and thymus (fig. 5.1).
4. Smile into your heart, feeling joy and love spread out from there to the lungs, liver, spleen, pancreas, kidneys, and genitals.

☯ Middle Line: The Digestive Tract

1. Bring smiling energy into the eyes, then down to the mouth.
2. Swallow saliva as you smile down to your stomach, small intestine (duodenum, jejunum, and ileum), large intestine (ascending colon, transverse colon, and descending colon), rectum, and anus (see fig. 5.2 on page 140).

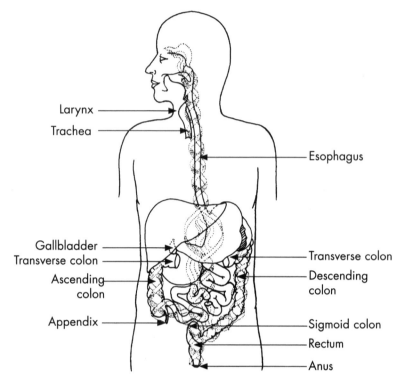

Fig. 5.2. Middle line smile: digestive tract

Back Line: The Governor Channel

1. Smile, and look upward about 3 inches into your mid-eyebrow point and pituitary gland.
2. Direct your smile to the Third Room, the small cavity deep in the center of your brain (fig. 5.3). Feel the room expand and grow with the bright golden light shining through the brain.
3. Smile into the thalamus, pineal gland (Crystal Room), and the left and right sides of the brain.
4. Smile to the midbrain and the brain stem, then to the base of your skull.
5. Smile down to the seven cervical vertebrae, the twelve thoracic vertebrae, the five lumbar vertebrae, then the sacrum and the tailbone.
6. Refresh the loving, soothing smile energy in your eyes, then smile

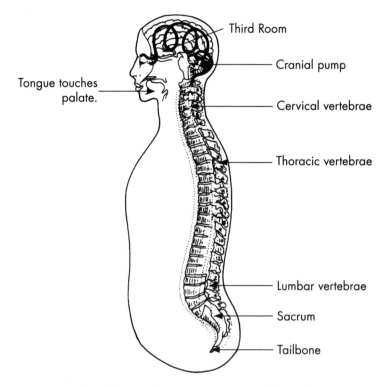

Third Room

Cranial pump

Tongue touches palate.

Cervical vertebrae

Thoracic vertebrae

Lumbar vertebrae

Sacrum

Tailbone

Fig. 5.3. Back line smile: Governor Channel

down the front, middle, and back lines in succession. Now do all of them at once, feeling bathed in a cooling waterfall or glowing sunshine of cosmic energy, smiles, joy, and love.

☯ Collect Energy in Navel

1. Gather all the smiling energy in your navel area—about 1½ inches inside your body. Spiral that energy with your mind or your hands from the center point to the outside. (Don't go above the diaphragm or below the pubic bone.)
2. Women spiral outward counterclockwise 36 times, then inward clockwise 24 times, returning energy toward the center. Finish by storing energy safely in the navel.

Microcosmic Orbit

1. After smiling down, collect the energy at the navel (fig. 5.4).
2. With the tongue touching the roof of the mouth, let the energy flow down to the sexual center.
3. Move the energy from the sexual center to the perineum.
4. Draw the energy up from the perineum to the sacrum.
5. Draw the energy up to the Ming Men, opposite the navel.
6. Draw the energy up to the T11 vertebrae.
7. Draw the energy up to the base of the skull.
8. Draw the energy up to the crown and circulate it.
9. Move the energy down from the crown to the mid-eyebrow.
10. Pass the energy down through the tongue to the throat center.
11. Bring the energy down from the throat to the heart center.
12. Bring the energy down to the solar plexus.
13. Bring the energy back to the navel.
14. Circulate the energy through this entire sequence at least 9 or 10 times.
15. Collect the energy at the navel. Cover your navel with both palms, right hand over left. Collect and mentally spiral the energy outward from the navel in a counterclockwise direction, making 36 revolutions. Once you have completed the counterclockwise revolutions, spiral the energy inward in a clockwise direction 24 times, ending and collecting the energy at the navel.

SIX HEALING SOUNDS

The Six Healing Sounds are produced subvocally and correspond to five specific organs: the lungs, kidneys, liver, heart, and spleen. The sixth sound is the "triple warmer," which evenly distributes energy throughout the body. Each sound creates its own energy to enhance and detoxify the internal system. All six sounds and their related postures decelerate the body after practice and remove excess heat accumulated in vital areas. A full description of this practice can be found in *The Six Healing Sounds* (Destiny Books, 2009).

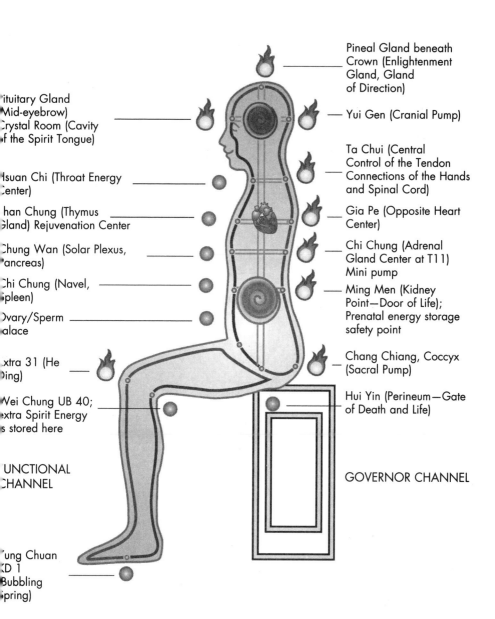

Pineal Gland beneath Crown (Enlightenment Gland, Gland of Direction)

Yui Gen (Cranial Pump)

Ta Chui (Central Control of the Tendon Connections of the Hands and Spinal Cord)

Gia Pe (Opposite Heart Center)

Chi Chung (Adrenal Gland Center at T11) Mini pump

Ming Men (Kidney Point—Door of Life); Prenatal energy storage safety point

Chang Chiang, Coccyx (Sacral Pump)

Hui Yin (Perineum—Gate of Death and Life)

GOVERNOR CHANNEL

Pituitary Gland (Mid-eyebrow) Crystal Room (Cavity of the Spirit Tongue)

Hsuan Chi (Throat Energy Center)

Shan Chung (Thymus Gland) Rejuvenation Center

Chung Wan (Solar Plexus, Pancreas)

Chi Chung (Navel, Spleen)

Ovary/Sperm Palace

Extra 31 (He Ding)

Wei Chung UB 40; Extra Spirit Energy is stored here

FUNCTIONAL CHANNEL

Yung Chuan KD 1 (Bubbling Spring)

Fig. 5.4. Energy circulating in the Microcosmic Orbit

Lung Exercise: The First Healing Sound

The lungs are associated with: the large intestine, the metal element, autumn, dryness, white color, pungent flavor, the nose, sense of smell, and the skin, as well as sadness, grief, courage, and justice.

1. While sitting in a chair with your eyes open, rest your hands—palms up—on your thighs.
2. Breathe in slowly and deeply and bring awareness to your lungs. Inhale and raise your arms until hands are at eye level, then rotate palms inward and continue to raise them above your head (fig. 5.5). Feel all along the arms into your shoulders, and feel the lungs and chest open.

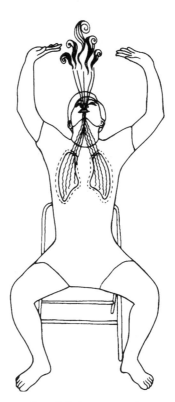

Fig. 5.5. Lung exercise

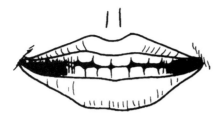

Fig. 5.6. Lungs' sound: sss-s-s-s-s-s

3. Close teeth and make the lungs' sound: "sss-s-s-s-s-s" slowly and evenly as you exhale (fig. 5.6). Picture the lungs exhaling a dark murky color, excess heat, and sick energy, sadness, sorrow, and grief.

4. Float palms down to lungs and then to your lap, facing up. Breathe in pure white light and the quality of righteousness. Close your eyes and smile to your lungs, imagining that you are still making the lungs' sound. Repeat these steps 3 to 6 times.

 ## Kidney Exercise: The Second Healing Sound

The kidneys are associated with: the urinary bladder, the water element, winter, cold, blue color, salty flavor, ears, hearing, and the bones, as well as fear and gentleness.

1. Breathe in slowly and deeply and bring awareness to your kidneys. Bend forward and clasp your hands together around your knees (see fig. 5.7 on page 146). Pull back on arms, feeling a stretch on your back, over the kidneys. Look up.

2. Round your lips and make the kidneys' sound: "choo-oo-oo-oo," while pulling your mid-abdomen in toward your spine (see fig. 5.8 on page 146). Blow out a dark murky color along with any excess heat, wet, sick energy, and fear.

3. Breathe in bright blue energy and the quality of gentleness. Separate your legs and rest your hands, palms up, on your thighs. Close your eyes and smile to your kidneys, imagining that you are still making the kidneys' sound. Repeat these steps 3 to 6 times.

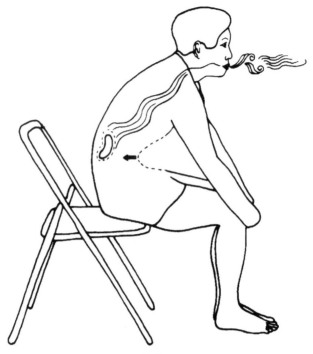

Fig. 5.7. Kidney exercise

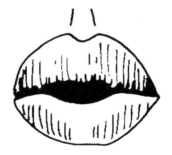

Fig. 5.8. Kidneys' sound: choo-oo-oo-oo

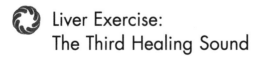 Liver Exercise:
The Third Healing Sound

The liver is associated with the gallbladder, the wood element, spring, moistness, the color green, the sour flavor, the eyes, and eyesight, as well as with anger, aggression, kindness, and forgiveness.

1. Breathe in slowly and deeply, becoming aware of the liver and its connection to the eyes. Beginning with your arms at your sides, palms out, slowly swing your arms up and over your head, following them with your eyes (fig. 5.9). Then interlace your fingers and push palms up toward the ceiling, feeling the stretch through arms and shoulders. Bend slightly to the left.

2. Open your eyes wide and exhale the sound "sh-h-h-h-h-h-h" subvocally (fig. 5.10), while breathing out a dark murky color filled with excess heat and anger.

3. Press the heels of your palms outward as you lower your shoulders, then place your hands in your lap, palms up. Breathe in a bright green energy and its quality of kindness. Let this energy fill your liver. Close your eyes and smile down to your liver. Repeat these steps 3 to 6 times.

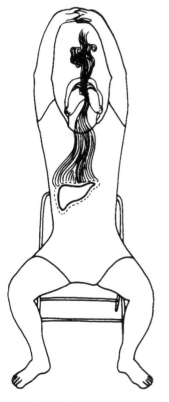

Fig. 5.9. Liver exercise

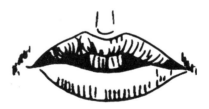

Fig. 5.10. Liver's sound: sh-h-h-h-h-h-h

🌀 Heart Exercise: The Fourth Healing Sound

The heart is associated with the small intestine, the fire element, summer, warmth, the color red, the bitter flavor, the tongue, and speech, as well as with joy, honor, love, creativity, and enthusiasm.

1. Breathe in slowly and deeply while focusing your awareness on your heart. Beginning with palms in your lap, inhale and swing your arms overhead, then clasp fingers together and push palms toward the ceiling, as in the liver exercise (fig. 5.11). This time, bend slightly to the right.

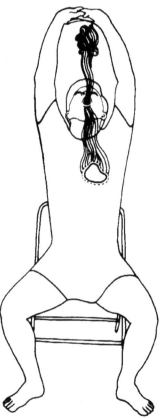

Fig. 5.11. Heart exercise

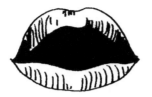

Fig. 5.12. Heart's sound: haw-w-w-w-w-w

2. Open your mouth, round your lips, and exhale the sound "haw-w-w-w-w-w" subvocally (fig. 5.12), while expelling dark murky energy along with any excess heat, impatience, arrogance, or cruelty.
3. Press palms outward and return hands to your lap, with palms facing upward. Breathe in bright red energy along with its qualities of joy, love, and respect. Smile down to your heart. Repeat these steps 3 to 6 times.

Spleen Exercise: The Fifth Healing Sound

The spleen is associated with the stomach and the pancreas, the earth element, Indian summer, dampness; the sweet flavor, the yellow color, the mouth, and taste, as well as with worry, compassion, balance, and openness.

1. Breathe in slowly and deeply, focusing your awareness on the spleen. Inhale and place the fingers of both hands beneath the left side of the rib cage, just below the sternum (see fig. 5.13 on page 150). Press your fingers inward as you push your middle back outward.
2. Exhale as you round your lips and make the sound of the spleen: "who-o-o-o-o-o" from your vocal cords (see fig. 5.14 on page 150). Expel any excess heat, dampness, worry, or pity.
3. Breathe a bright yellow light into your spleen, stomach, and pancreas, filling them with fairness, compassion, and centeredness. Lower your hands slowly to your lap, palms up, and smile down to your spleen. Repeat these steps 3 to 6 times.

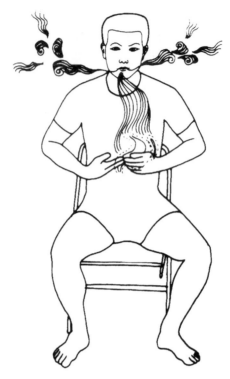

Fig. 5.13. Spleen exercise

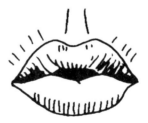

Fig. 5.14. Spleen's sound: who-o-o-o-o-o

 Triple Warmer Exercise:
The Sixth Healing Sound

The triple warmer consists of the upper warmer (hot: includes the brain, neck, thymus, heart, lungs), the middle warmer (warm: includes the liver, stomach, and spleen), and the lower warmer (cool: includes the intestines, kidneys, and genitals).

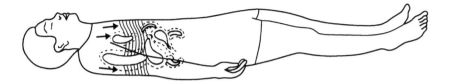

Fig. 5.15. Triple Warmer exercise

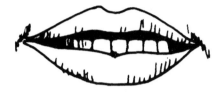

Fig. 5.16. Triple Warmer's sound: hee-e-e-e-e-e

1. Lie on your back, close your eyes, and take a deep breath (fig. 5.15). Inhale fully into all three heaters.
2. Exhale with the sound "hee-e-e-e-e-e" made subvocally (fig. 5.16). Imagine a large roller pressing out your breath from the top of your chest and rolling down toward your lower abdomen. Imagine your chest and abdomen are flat-feeling light, bright, and empty.
3. Rest by breathing normally, then repeat these steps 3 to 6 times.

OVARIAN BREATHING AND COMPRESSION

These two Healing Love practices rechannel sexual energy to heal the internal system. Full descriptions can be found in *Bone Marrow Nei Kung* (Destiny Books, 2006) and *Healing Love through the Tao* (Destiny Books, 2005).

 Ovarian Breathing

1. Sit with your vagina and perineum unconstricted, with no drafts, or sit on ball against the clitoris; palms on knees; chin tucked in. Or stand, hands at sides; feet shoulder-width apart.

2. Place both thumbs on the navel and use your index fingers to form a triangle. The place where the index fingers touch is the Ovarian Palace. Spread out your little fingers evenly: underneath the points where they rest are the ovaries. Breathe into the ovaries.
3. Rub the ovaries as you use the PC muscle to open and close the vagina; inhale and bring energy from the ovaries to the Ovarian Palace; exhale.
4. Inhale and pull the energy of the ovaries to the Ovarian Palace, then down to the perineum; retain the energy there; exhale. Repeat 9 times.
5. Inhale as you collect the energy from the ovaries in the Ovarian Palace, then pull it down to the perineum, and from there up to the sacrum. Hold the attention at the sacrum and exhale slowly. Repeat 9 times.
6. Inhale and guide the energy from the ovaries to the Ovarian Palace to the perineum and through the sacrum up to T11 in the same manner, then relax and exhale. Repeat 9 times. Repeat the process 9 times at each of the following stations in turn: C7, Jade Pillow at the base of the skull, and crown.
7. At the crown, spiral the energy in your brain 9 to 36 times counterclockwise, then 9 to 36 times clockwise. With your tongue on your palate, allow the energy to flow down to the third eye, tongue, throat, heart, solar plexus, and the navel. Collect the energy at the navel.

Ovarian Compression

1. Sit on the edge of a chair, feet flat on the floor, or stand, hands at sides; feet shoulder-width apart.
2. Inhale deeply and compress the energy into an imaginary energy (chi) ball at the solar plexus; roll it down to navel, pelvic region, and the ovaries.
3. Compress air into the ovaries and down into the vagina for as long as you can. Contract the lips of the vagina tightly, squeeze the anus, and tighten the perineum to prevent energy loss.

4. While maintaining the compression, keep your tongue pressed against your palate; swallow deeply into the sexual center.
5. Exhale and relax. Rest by taking quick, shallow breaths through the nose. Relax by rotating the waist with arms at shoulder level several times.
6. Repeat 9 to 18 times morning and evening.

BONE BREATHING
AND BONE COMPRESSION

Bones are extremely porous, and they are always "breathing." The pores allow the passage of oxygen, blood, and nutrition through the bones in the same way a sponge absorbs and releases water. Bone Breathing draws external chi into the bones through the skin, muscles, and tendons. After external energy has been breathed into a particular area, Bone Compression is used to force the combined energies into the bones to burn the fat out of the marrow, thereby assisting in the marrow's regeneration. Step-by-step detailed instructions for the performance of Bone Breathing and Bone Compression, along with further information regarding their health benefits, can be found in *Bone Marrow Nei Kung* (Destiny Books, 2006).

While Bone Breathing is a mental process used in conjunction with long, soft breath cycles, Bone Compression is a physical process of contracting the muscles, thereby squeezing chi into the bones. This energy is used to complement previously stored sexual energy, which is released into the body through the Sexual Energy Massage or Chi Weight Lifting.

The techniques should initially be practiced from a seated position.

 ## Bone Breathing

Before beginning the Bone Breathing exercise, you should first be certain that the Microcosmic Orbit is clear of any blockages. Regulate your breathing, then circulate your energy through the Microcosmic Orbit for several cycles.

1. Create a sensation of coolness in the fingers of either hand. Inhale, and draw warm external energies into that hand through the fingers. Apply this to the opposite hand. Exhale, and release the energy.

2. Pull up your perineum region slightly as you breathe chi further up into the ulna and radius bones of the lower arm. Practice first on each arm, then on both together. Exhale, and release.

3. Apply the same procedure to the upper arms, drawing chi to the humerus bones. Exhale, and release the energy. Remember to draw energy in with more force with each new inhalation, thereby accessing further points within each limb.

4. Draw chi up through the scapulae and collarbone to reach the C7 point and the cranium but do not leave it there. Either combine it at T11 with the energy drawn from the legs or store it in the navel.

5. Create a sensation of coolness in the toes of either foot. Inhale and draw the warm external energies into that foot through the toes. Apply this to the opposite foot. Exhale, and release the energy.

6. Pull up your perineum region slightly as you breathe chi further up into the tibia and fibula bones of the lower legs. If necessary, practice on each leg individually, and then draw chi into both legs together. Exhale, and release.

7. With each breath, draw the chi further up into the femur bones of the upper legs, into the hips, and then to the sacrum. Exhale, but retain the energy you have breathed into these areas.

8. If you choose to combine the procedures for the arms and legs, do not draw the energy to the skull from the arms directly, but instead combine it with the energy from the legs at the center of the spine. First breathe into both hands and feet simultaneously. Inhale chi all the way up to the shoulders and scapulae through the arms, and up to the thigh and hip bones through the legs. Combine this energy at the middle of the spine after it has reached the sacrum and the scapulae from their respective sources. From the center of the spine, move the energy up to the head, and then back down the spine to where the ribs begin. Exhale as needed.

9. Breathe the energy outward through the twelve ribs, encompassing the rib cage from the front to the back, and recombine the chi at the sternum. Breathe into the sternum. Exhale.

Bone Compression

1. Use the same steps as in Bone Breathing, but retain the chi by spiraling it throughout the limbs. Inhale, pulling up the perineum region, then spiral the energy up from the fingers and toes throughout the arms and legs to meet at the center of the spine.
2. Having combined the external energy drawn from both sources at the center of the spine, expand the chi outward through the twelve ribs, spiraling it into the sternum.
3. The body's capacity has been reached when you can no longer spiral new chi into the arms. Begin to pack the chi, condensing it into the same space as the energy that has been accumulated.
4. Contract the muscles of the hands and arms with each breath. Hold the breath with each contraction.
5. Exhale as you release the contraction. When you release your hold, use your mind to absorb energy into the bones through the pores of the skin. During resting periods, the sensation of drawing in energy through the skin should be felt throughout the body. Bones, muscles, and tendons should begin to feel as though they are wrapped in cotton.
6. After you have practiced for a while, feel the sensation inside your bones. If you have a lot of fat, the feeling will be very hot. This is the fat beginning to melt.
7. It is a good idea to practice with the tongue on the palate because the energy will begin to move through the Microcosmic Orbit; touching the tongue to the roof of the mouth enables the energy to flow in a circle up the spine and down the front of the body.

INCREASING CHI
AND KIDNEY PRESSURE

These two practices, presented in chapter 3, should precede the Power Lock and Chi Weight Lifting. A full description can be found in *Bone Marrow Nei Kung* (Destiny Books, 2006).

 ## Increasing Chi Pressure

1. Place the middle finger of each hand about 1½ inches below the navel at the lower tan tien.
2. Concentrate on the lower tan tien as you inhale chi into it, expanding the point with the resulting pressure.

 ## Increasing Kidney Pressure

1. Stand in a Horse stance with your feet slightly wider than shoulder width. Rub your hands together until they are warm, and then apply their warmth to the kidneys by placing your energized palms on them from the back.
2. Bend your upper body forward slightly as you inhale, and pull up the left and right sides of the anus as you draw chi up to the kidneys.
3. Exhale, and deflate the kidneys.
4. Follow this sequence up to 36 times, and finish by warming the hands and again placing them on the kidneys.

POWER LOCK

More detail on this practice can be found in chapter 1 of this book and in *Bone Marrow Nei Kung* (Destiny Books, 2006). The Power Lock should be practiced before and after the Sexual Energy Massage.

Power Lock

1. Begin with Ovarian Breathing, slightly contracting the vagina to accumulate Ching Chi in the Ovarian Palace.

2. Use short inhalations to draw the energy from the Ovarian Palace through each successive point leading up to the first station: inhale a sip of air and contract the perineum, drawing the energy there; then inhale again as you contract the anus and draw the energy there; then with the next sip of air, pull up the back part of the anus as you draw the energy up to the sacrum. Use your fingers to press on the perineum point each time you inhale and contract, releasing them briefly before each subsequent contraction. Use 9 contractions with 9 sips of air to draw Ching Chi from the Ovarian Palace to the sacrum. Hold the energy at the sacrum as you exhale and return your attention to the Ovarian Palace.

3. Repeat this entire sequence for each subsequent station: T11, C7, Jade Pillow, and the crown.

4. Spiral the energy at the crown 9 to 36 times outward, then inward.

5. Bring the energy down and store it in the navel.

CLOTH MASSAGE, SEXUAL ENERGY MASSAGE, AND INTERNAL EGG EXERCISE

The Sexual Energy Massage and Internal Egg Exercise are preceded by the Cloth Massage to activate Ching Chi. Below are summaries of the practices presented in chapter 2 of this book. A full description of these practices can be found in *Bone Marrow Nei Kung* (Destiny Books, 2006).

 Preparation: Cloth Massage

Massage the mons, labial area, and vaginal muscles, then, in turn, the perineum, the coccyx, and the sacrum with a silk cloth. Spiral at each location 36 times clockwise and 36 times counterclockwise. Feel enlarged breasts and moist vagina.

Sexual Energy Massage

Rub your hands together briskly to warm them up before performing each of the following steps, which together make chi comprised of energy from the organs, the glands, and the sexual center available for your practice.

1. Breast Massage: Sit naked or loosely clothed, with some pressure on the vagina. Pull up the middle and back parts of the anus, drawing the chi up the spinal cord. Pull up the left and right sides of the anus, bringing the chi into your nipples. Place the second joint of the middle fingers on your nipples. Place your tongue on the roof of your mouth.

2. Massaging the Glands with Accumulated Chi: Place three fingers on each breast and circle outward from the nipples—clockwise for the right hand, and counterclockwise for the left hand. Then circle inward. Repeat the outward and inward circles with the right hand moving counterclockwise and the left hand moving clockwise. Continue massaging as you draw chi to the pituitary gland, then return that chi to the breasts. Repeat this process with the thyroid and parathyroid glands, thymus gland, pancreas, and adrenal glands, each time bringing the energy back to the breasts.

3. Massaging the Organs with Accumulated Chi: Place your hands on your breasts. Let the chi from the thymus and the breasts activate the chi of the lungs, then return that chi to the breasts. Direct the accumulated chi to activate the heart, then return it to the breasts, and repeat this process with the spleen, kidneys, and liver. Then place your palms on your knees and focus attention on your breasts, letting energy expand into the nipples, then flow down into the ovaries. Breathe directly into the ovaries as you lightly move the lips of the vagina open and closed. Merge energy from both ovaries and concentrate in the Ovarian Palace as you squeeze the genital area in slightly.

4. Massaging the Ovaries: Place your fingertips on your ovaries and massage them in small circles—36 times clockwise and 36 times counterclockwise.

Internal Egg Exercise

1. Insert the egg into your vagina large end first. Stand in Horse stance and tightly contract the muscles that close the vaginal orifice to hold the egg in the vaginal canal.
2. Inhale and contract the muscles immediately in front of your cervix while keeping the first set of muscles contracted.
3. Using the muscles in the middle of the vaginal canal, lightly squeeze the egg. Inhale and squeeze harder, then move the egg up and down. When you are out of breath, exhale and rest.
4. Use the top set of muscles—those in front of the cervix—to move the egg left and right, then rest. Now use the bottom set of muscles (controlling the vaginal orifice) to move the egg left and right.
5. Use the top set of muscles, then the bottom set, to tilt the egg up and down. Combine all of the movements, then slide the egg up to touch the cervix, and down to the vaginal orifice. Release.
6. Increase the speed of motion until you feel the need to rest. Take a deep breath and draw the accumulated energy into the Microcosmic Orbit.
7. Remove the egg and do the Cloth Massage.
8. Rest and practice the healing sounds of the lung and heart and the Microcosmic Orbit.

CHI WEIGHT LIFTING WITH PREPARATORY AND CONCLUDING PRACTICES

We wish to remind our readers that Chi Weight Lifting is included in this text for the documentation of its procedure as a guide for instructors and trained students of the Universal Healing Tao. It is not intended for beginning students. Universal Healing Tao cannot and will not be held responsible for any reader of this book who attempts Chi Weight Lifting without first receiving qualified instruction. A more extensive description can be found in *Bone Marrow Nei Kung* (Destiny Books, 2006).

Preparation for Chi Weight Lifting

To maintain safety, Chi Weight Lifting should always be done after doing the following exercises:

1. Increasing Chi Pressure: Practice from 9 to 81 times.
2. Increasing Kidney Pressure: Practice from 6 to 36 times.
3. Power Lock Exercise: 2 to 3 times up to the crown.
4. Cloth Massage of sexual center, perineum, and sacrum.
5. Sexual Energy Massage:
   a. Breast Massage
   b. Massage the Glands with Accumulated Chi
   c. Massage the Organs with Accumulated Chi
   d. Massage the Ovaries
6. Internal Egg Exercise (optional)

Chi Weight Lifting

1. Prepare the weight on the floor or a chair. (After inserting the string through the egg, tie it to the weight or the weight-lifting apparatus.)
2. Insert the egg into the vagina, larger end first.
3. Hold the weight with your hands while standing up to assume the Horse stance. While testing the weight with your index and middle fingers, inhale as you contract the anus and perineum, then contract and hold first the lower and then the middle and upper vaginal muscles, so that the egg pushes deeply up into the vaginal canal.
4. If the weight does not feel too heavy, gently release the string from the fingers, until you are holding the weight with the contracted muscles of the vagina. Pull up from the cervix.
5. When you feel you are holding the egg and the weight securely, swing the weight from 36 to 60 times, inhaling as you pull up with each forward swing. Exhale as the weight moves backward.
6. Lift the weight from each station of the Microcosmic Orbit: sacrum, Door of Life, T11, C7, base of the skull, Crown point, third eye, and

let it flow down the front channel; collect the energy at the navel.

7. Rest as you hold the weight manually, or place it on a raised surface, such as a chair. (You may prefer to remove it while resting, and then attach it again to resume lifting.)

8. Gently release the weight between your legs once again to lift it with the power of the organs and glands, starting with the kidneys.

10. Lower the weight to the chair or the floor, and then remove the egg.

Concluding Exercises

1. Power Lock Exercise: 2 to 3 times up to the crown.

2. Cloth Massage of the sexual center, perineum, and sacrum.

3. Sexual Energy Massage.

4. Use at least two or three of the Six Healing Sounds, especially the heart and lung sounds. All of them are useful if you have the time to do them.

5. Practice the Microcosmic Orbit meditation for several minutes. In conjunction with this meditation, you can also practice Bone Breathing. Use your mind to absorb the released Ching Chi into the bones.

With these practices of Chi Kung for women's health and sexual vitality you now have the opportunity to heal and balance yourself. May the Tao be with you.

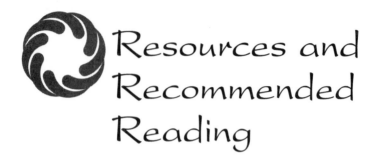

Resources and Recommended Reading

In this section we have listed several sources for the cleansing supplements and colonic supplies that we have recommended in the book, as well as more information on acid and alkaline balance in the diet and recommended nutritional supplements. In addition, a list of books for recommended reading will guide your further study of the topics covered in this book.

CLEANSING SUPPLEMENTS AND COLONIC SUPPLIES

Bernard Jensen International
1255 Linda Vista Drive
San Marcos, CA 92078
Phone: 760-471-9977
Fax: 760-471-9989
E-mail: info@bernardjensen.com
Website: www.bernardjensen.com

Bernard Jensen International carries a wide variety of natural supplements and detoxifying products including colonic boards and supplies. We have listed a few of their supplements below, but see their website for the full range of products.

Niacin

Niacin or nicotinic acid, a water-soluble B-complex vitamin and anti-hyperlipidemic agent, is 3-pyridinecarboxylic acid. It is a white, crystalline powder, sparingly soluble in water. Niacin is essential in energy production at the cellular level. Niacin helps maintain proper metabolic function. Niacin is used for lowering the levels of LDL ("bad") cholesterol or of triglyceride in the blood of certain patients. It may be used in combination with diet or other medicines. It may also be used for other conditions as determined by your doctor. It works by decreasing the amount of a certain protein that is necessary for the formation of cholesterol in the body.

Nova Scotia Dulse (Dulse Tablets)

Nova Scotia Dulse is a sea vegetable that is a natural source of essential vitamins, ions, sea salt, and roughage. Harvested from the cold waters of the North Atlantic, this premium dulse is then sun-dried to preserve the natural nutrients. Each tablet provides you with a variety of essential vitamins, minerals, protein, and trace elements the way nature intended. These tablets give you the sodium necessary to assist in moving the waste from the cells in a cellular cleanse.

Vitamin C

This natural source vitamin C tablet contains natural vitamin C derived from dehydrated juice of the acerola berry and wild Spanish orange. These food sources provide the vitamin C complex (i.e., bioflavonoids and other synergistic nutrients), factors not present in supplements that use ascorbic acid (chemical form of vitamin C). This vitamin C has a 100 mg equivalent of ascorbic acid per serving, supplying 110 percent of the Recommended Daily Allowance (RDA). Because vitamin C is constantly being utilized, it should be taken in small repeated doses throughout the day. Chewable tablets are ideal for this purpose, providing easy and rapid absorption of the natural vitamin C complex.

Colema Boards of California, Inc.
P.O. Box 1879
Cottonwood, CA 96022
Toll free: 800-745-2446
Phone: 530-347-5700
Fax: 530-347-2336
E-mail: info@colema.com
Website: www.colema.com

The best source for genuine Colema colonic boards, tubing, and supplies. This company also carries a wide variety of supplements and colonic cleansing products.

V. E. Irons, Inc.
P.O. Box 34710
North Kansas City, MO 64116
Toll free: 800-544-8147
Phone: 816-221-3719
Fax: 816-221-1272
E-mail: info@veirons.com
Website: www.veirons.com

V. E. Irons is home of Vit-Ra-Tox Products and manufacturers of quality whole food supplements since 1946. We have listed several products available from V. E. Irons below, but see their website for the full product line.

Detoxificant (Bentonite)
This substance is a natural and powerful detoxificant derived from bentonite, a mineral-rich volcanic clay. The active detoxifying ingredient is montmorillonite ("mont-mor-ill-o-nite"). Montmorillonite possesses the ability to adsorb about forty times its own weight in positively charged substances present in the alimentary canal. Because montmorillonite has such strong adsorptive properties and is not digested, it tightly binds material to be excreted. It is a perfect accompaniment to the Intestinal Cleanser (see p. 165). Mixed together in juice, this

cleansing drink offers the scrubbing and roughage benefits from soluble and insoluble fiber from psyllium, and the detoxification properties of bentonite.

Intestinal Cleanser (Psyllium)

Intestinal Cleanser is a finely ground powder of imported psyllium husk and seed. As it contains primarily fiber and no laxative or herbal stimulants, it can be used on a daily basis to assist normal bowel peristalsis. Psyllium has a hydrophilic (water-loving) action that softens hardened mucus lining the bowel wall, facilitating its elimination. The Intestinal Cleanser and Detoxificant are ideal companion products to be used together for maximum alimentary canal detoxification.

Fasting Plus (Enzyme Supplement)

Never before has the use of antacids and gastric medication to treat indigestion been so prevalent. These types of drugs block the body's natural digestive processes, but this enzymatic supplement aids the digestion process by providing natural digestive enzymes to break down food and promote assimilation of nutrients. Each tablet contains two layers of digestive enzymes. The outer portion contains pepsin, which digests protein into soluble amino acids, proteases, and peptones. Pepsin is activated by the low pH of the stomach, so people suspected of gastric acid deficiency would benefit from it. The inner portion of the tablet becomes activated in the small intestine and contains natural digestive agents: bovine bile salts that promote absorption of lipids and activate pancreatic lipase (a fat-digesting enzyme), and the pancreatic substances amylase (for starch) and proteases (for protein), plus tyrosine, chymotrypsin, and other proteolytic enzymes. Because the inner portion is intended to work in the intestine, the tablets should be swallowed whole.

GreenLife (Chlorophyll Gel Capsules)

GreenLife is a 100 percent vegetable food containing 92 percent dried extracted juices of organically grown cereal grasses: barley, oats, rye, and wheat (no chemical fertilizers or insecticides are used); and 8 percent papain, beets, and sea kelp. The grasses are cut at the young, rapidly growing stage, when the maximum nutrition is in the blade. GreenLife is a concentrated product, retaining its natural balance as a complete all-food supplement. It is nontoxic in any consumable amount and helps balance nutritional deficiencies resulting from consumption of devitalized and processed foods.

Pro-Gest (Vegetarian Pancreatic Enzymes)

The active ingredient in Pro-Gest is papain, which is derived from the papaya fruit. Papain is a natural proteolytic enzyme that breaks down proteins and supports a healthy digestive process. Other ingredients include papaya seed meal, Russian black radish, and betaine hydrochloride in a base of dried juice from organically grown beets—the same powder used for Whole Beet Plant Juice Tablets (see below). The betaine hydrochloride acts to supplement the natural hydrochloric acid in the stomach.

Wheat Germ Oil/Flaxseed Oil

The wheat germ oil capsules contain 73 percent wheat germ oil, an excellent source of the natural vitamin E complex; and 27 percent flaxseed oil, a rich source of unsaturated, essential fatty acids including: alpha linolenic acid, omega-6, and omega-3. Vitamin E is an essential dietary component that is necessary for antioxidant activity in membranes. It regenerates other cellular antioxidants (i.e., selenium and glutathione) after they become oxidized. The essential fatty acids also must be obtained in the diet and are precursors for many hormones and metabolically active compounds. The natural vitamin E in our foods is destroyed during cooking and processing due to heat, light, air, and freezing. Grains lose up to 80 percent of their vitamin E content when milled. Commercially processed vegetable oils are low in vitamin E. It has become quite clear that there is a need for natural vitamin E supplementation in our modern diets.

Whole Beet Plant Juice Tablets

The beets used for this product are organically grown. The whole beet (leaves, stems, and root) is juiced, and the extract is vacuum dried at low temperature to retain maximum quantities of the enzymes, vitamins, and mineral factors. Unlike inorganic sources of iron, the body assimilates iron from the beetroot very easily, because iron is found in an organic complex. Beets also contain potassium, magnesium, phosphorous, calcium, sulfur, iodine, vitamins, and many trace minerals.

PH BALANCED DIET

Website: www.thealkalinediet.org
Provides extensive information about acid/alkaline balance, food lists, and resources for further information.

Website: www.trans4mind.com/nutrition/pH.html
Includes a how-to on urine and saliva testing, food charts, and a look at the science behind acid/alkaline food chemistry.

RECOMMENDED READING

Chia, Mantak. *The Alchemy of Sexual Energy.* Rochester, Vt.: Destiny Books, 2009.
———. *Bone Marrow Nei Kung.* Rochester, Vt.: Destiny Books, 2006.
———. *Chi Self-Massage.* Rochester, Vt.: Destiny Books, 2006.
———. *Cosmic Detox.* Rochester, Vt.: Destiny Books, 2011.
———. *Healing Love through the Tao.* Rochester, Vt.: Destiny Books, 2005.
———. *The Inner Smile.* Rochester, Vt.: Destiny Books, 2008.
———. *Iron Shirt Chi Kung.* Rochester, Vt.: Destiny Books, 2006.
———. *The Six Healing Sounds.* Rochester, Vt.: Destiny Books, 2009.
———. *Wisdom Chi Kung.* Rochester, Vt.: Destiny Books, 2008.
Chia, Mantak, and William U. Wei. *Basic Practices of the Universal Healing Tao.* Rochester, Vt.: Destiny Books, 2013.
———. *Cosmic Nutrition.* Rochester, Vt.: Destiny Books, 2012.
———. *Sexual Reflexology.* Rochester, Vt.: Destiny Books, 2003.

Primack, Jeff. *Conquering Any Disease.* Sunny Isles Beach, Fla.: Press On Qi Productions, 2008.

———. *Smoothie Formulas.* Sunny Isles Beach, Fla.: Press On Qi Productions, 2008.

Stanchion, Lino. *Power Eating Program.* Asheville, N.C.: Healthy Products, Inc., 1989.

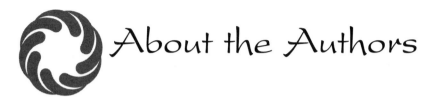 # About the Authors

MANTAK CHIA

Mantak Chia has been studying the Taoist approach to life since childhood. His mastery of this ancient knowledge, enhanced by his study of other disciplines, has resulted in the development of the Universal Healing Tao system, which is now being taught throughout the world.

Mantak Chia was born in Thailand to Chinese parents in 1944. When he was six years old, he learned from Buddhist monks how to sit and "still the mind." While in grammar school he learned traditional Thai boxing, and he soon went on to acquire considerable skill in aikido, yoga, and Tai Chi. His studies of the Taoist way of life began in earnest when he was a student in Hong Kong, ultimately leading to his mastery of a wide variety of esoteric disciplines, with the guidance of several masters, including Master I Yun, Master Meugi, Master Cheng Yao Lun, and Master Pan Yu. To better understand the mechanisms behind healing energy, he also studied Western anatomy and medical sciences.

Master Chia has taught his system of healing and energizing practices to tens of thousands of students and trained more than two thousand instructors and practitioners throughout the world. He has established centers for Taoist study and training in many countries around the globe. In June of 1990, he was honored by the International Congress of Chinese Medicine and Qi Gong (Chi Kung), which named him the Qi Gong Master of the Year.

WILLIAM U. WEI

Born after World War II, growing up in the Midwest area of the United States, and trained in Catholicism, William Wei became a student of the Tao under Master Mantak Chia in the early 1980s. In the later 1980s he became a senior instructor of the Universal Healing Tao, specializing in one-on-one training. In the early 1990s William Wei moved to Tao Garden, Thailand, and assisted Master Mantak Chia in building Tao Garden Taoist Training Center. For six years William traveled to over thirty countries, teaching with Master Mantak Chia and serving as marketing and construction coordinator for the Tao Garden. Upon completion of Tao Garden in December 2000, he became project manager for all the Universal Tao Publications and products. With the purchase of a mountain with four waterfalls in southern Oregon, USA, in the late 1990s, William Wei is presently completing a Taoist Mountain Sanctuary for personal cultivation, higher-level practices, and ascension. William Wei is the coauthor with Master Chia of *Sexual Reflexology, Living in the Tao,* and the Taoist poetry book of 366 daily poems, *Emerald River,* which expresses the feeling, essence, and stillness of the Tao. William U. Wei, also known as Wei Tzu, is a pen name for this instructor so the instructor can remain anonymous and can continue to become a blade of grass in a field of grass.

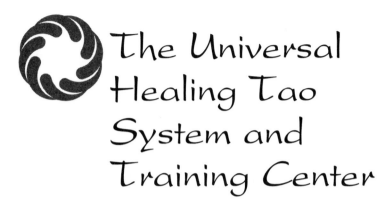

The Universal Healing Tao System and Training Center

THE UNIVERSAL HEALING TAO SYSTEM

The ultimate goal of Taoist practice is to transcend physical boundaries through the development of the soul and the spirit within the human. That is also the guiding principle behind the Universal Healing Tao, a practical system of self-development that enables individuals to complete the harmonious evolution of their physical, mental, and spiritual bodies. Through a series of ancient Chinese meditative and internal energy exercises, the practitioner learns to increase physical energy, release tension, improve health, practice self-defense, and gain the ability to heal him- or herself and others. In the process of creating a solid foundation of health and well-being in the physical body, the practitioner also creates the basis for developing his or her spiritual potential by learning to tap in to the natural energies of the sun, moon, earth, stars, and other environmental forces.

The Universal Healing Tao practices are derived from ancient techniques rooted in the processes of nature. They have been gathered and integrated into a coherent, accessible system for well-being that works directly with the life force, or chi, that flows through the meridian system of the body.

Master Chia has spent years developing and perfecting techniques for teaching these traditional practices to students around the world through ongoing classes, workshops, private instruction, and healing sessions, as well as books and video and audio products. Further information can be obtained at www.universal-tao.com.

THE UNIVERSAL HEALING TAO TRAINING CENTER

The Tao Garden Resort and Training Center in northern Thailand is the home of Master Chia and serves as the worldwide headquarters for Universal Healing Tao activities. This integrated wellness, holistic health, and training center is situated on eighty acres surrounded by the beautiful Himalayan foothills near the historic walled city of Chiang Mai. The serene setting includes flower and herb gardens ideal for meditation, open-air pavilions for practicing Chi Kung, and a health and fitness spa.

The center offers classes year round, as well as summer and winter retreats. It can accommodate two hundred students, and group leasing can be arranged. For information on courses, books, products, and other Universal Healing Tao resources, see below.

Universal Healing Tao Center
274 Moo 7, Luang Nua, Doi Saket, Chiang Mai, 50220 Thailand
Tel: (66)(53) 495-596 Fax: (66)(53) 495-852
E-mail: universaltao@universal-tao.com
Web site: www.universal-tao.com

For information on retreats and the health spa, contact:

Tao Garden Health Spa and Resort
E-mail: info@tao-garden.com, taogarden@hotmail.com
Web site: www.tao-garden.com

Good Chi • Good Heart • Good Intention

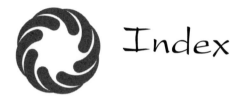

Index

Page numbers in *italics* refer to illustrations.

BOOKS OF RELATED INTEREST

Healing Love through the Tao
Cultivating Female Sexual Energy
by Mantak Chia

Sexual Reflexology
Activating the Taoist Points of Love
by Mantak Chia and William U. Wei

Karsai Nei Tsang
Therapeutic Massage for the Sexual Organs
by Mantak Chia

Taoist Foreplay
Love Meridians and Pressure Points
by Mantak Chia and Kris Deva North

Healing Light of the Tao
Foundational Practices to Awaken Chi Energy
by Mantak Chia

Chi Self-Massage
The Taoist Way of Rejuvenation
by Mantak Chia

The Sexual Teachings of the White Tigress
Secrets of the Female Taoist Masters
by Hsi Lai

The Estrogen Alternative
A Guide to Natural Hormonal Balance
by Raquel Martin and Judi Gerstung, D.C.

INNER TRADITIONS • BEAR & COMPANY
P.O. Box 388
Rochester, VT 05767
1-800-246-8648
www.InnerTraditions.com

Or contact your local bookseller